D0563525

Suddenly Skinny: A Weight Loss Survival Guide

How to lose a ton of weight and how to cope with it when you do.

Freya Taylor

Copyright © 2011 Freya Taylor

All rights reserved.

ISBN: 1466331569
ISBN-13: 978-1466331563

DEDICATION

Dedicated to the most wonderful, strong, compassionate formerly fat women anywhere—my friends from the Medifast discussion boards: Chris, Chatty, De, Corbie, Connor, Serafina, and so many others who encouraged me and kicked my ass with relentless Tough Love. All errors and misinformation are my own. Anything I got right I probably owe to them.

I also can't thank enough my dear friend Kathleen. Without your support, encouragement, blunt honesty, fashion advice, shopping tutorials, and companionship, I would be a lesser person. You taught me to always be as pretty as possible for destiny.

CONTENTS

FREYA TAYLOR

INTRODUCTION

I'm a bit intense about making a real, lasting change in your life, because I believe you can. *I believe you can.* I believe you can have health, a bounce in your step, the freedom to wear the size clothes you want to wear, and a whole new joy in your life. Because I believe in you, I don't hold back. I tell it like it is, because I know that along your road to a radically changed life, you are going to dive into the hard work and you need the truth for that.

Is this book for you?

It's not the right book for you if you want soft, fluffy bunny words like "just listen to your body" (your body is an entitled greedy lying brat, and listening to it is why you're fat), "you're only human," or any other enabling nonsense.

This book is not for you if you just want to take off ten vanity pounds to look better in your bikini. This book is for women who may never wear a bikini again, but who still want to be able to rock their look in clothes and run around with their grandkids.

This book is not for you if you want to lose weight for your wedding and then balloon back up as soon as the ring is on and the fat management garment is off.

Is this book for you if you're male? Most people who admit to dieting are chicks. Sorry, gentlemen, but you're under-represented in the weight-loss book-buying public. I have written this book with a mostly female audience in mind. However, if you can tolerate my breezy girl-talk tone and use of the feminine pronoun, almost all of the information in here is useful for anyone losing weight, regardless of gender.

Who is it for? This book is for people who are overweight, who want to change their lives *for good*.

That's a daunting task. And it's made harder because all the weight loss info out there focuses on only half of the equation—how to take the weight off. Nobody spends any time telling you how not to freak out when your entire life is upended by this radical change. People regain their weight only partly because they have unresolved food issues. It's also partly because they're used to a certain status quo, and not given any direction for how to handle life as a thin person.

Everyone seems to think that the story ends when you win the lottery. They hand you a check, you buy a bunch of cool stuff, and you live happily ever after. Likewise, you get thin, you are issued your size six jeans, and you drive off into the sunset with your perfect life.

Elements of truth exist in the fantasy—yes, it's amazing getting thin. I imagine it's amazing winning the lottery, too, but if you ask me which I'd prefer, I'll tell you thin and working for a living beats fat and any amount of money.

I'm here to help you with both parts of the equation. Getting thin, and living with it once you do. This book is a comprehensive look at the physical, mental, and emotional aspects of losing weight, as well as a how-to guide for coping with the physical, style, lifestyle, social, romantic, and eating changes getting thin will bring. It will revolutionize your world.

Are you ready?

Bring it. I want to see you *HOT.*

I. WHO AM I TO TALK?

I lost a hundred pounds. I went from 235 pounds in a size twenty-four to 135 pounds in a size six. I lost eighteen inches *each* off my waist and hips. I did it in nine months and twenty-five days.

I was fat since childhood, and no matter how thin I am on the outside there's a part of me that's sure I'll make one wrong move and wake up in the morning with the fat girl back on the outside again. And yet? When I wake up in the morning I now pull on size six jeans, no matter how long I was fat before.

How did I get from there to here?

I first remember knowing I was fat around fifth grade. I wasn't huge, but a little goes a long way when other children are quick to mock any difference. Why was I fat? Endless reasons... Emotional trauma, absorbing my mother's own struggle with food and weight, food was used as a "treat" or a break from work, I ate to stuff my feelings, I used the weight to hide from male attention, the crappy suburban American diet of the 70's and 80's, a sedentary family, etc. I had my reasons.

My reasons stayed with me, and collected new reasons. When you're used to relying on something as an emotional crutch, it's a hard habit to break. My weight would go up for a while, then down, then back up. During my adult life, it was 50 pounds a breakup. I did this three times before I realized it was a pattern I needed to change or I would be fat forever. Because I didn't take 50 pounds back off every time, and my trend was steadily upwards.

I was a success and a failure on every diet I ever tried. I was a success because once I decided to lose weight and started a diet, I did lose weight. I would take off 30 pounds or so and start feeling great. I'd be full of energy, loving the way I was looking in my clothes, and I'd drift right back off the diet. I had no problem with that, actually. So what if I weighed 170? I felt fit, full of life, and had a new boyfriend. Every diet was a success.

But then the last breakup was harder. Really, *really* hard. I just didn't stop eating. I ate my misery all the way up to 235 pounds and a size 24. It was interfering with my life. I didn't want to move around, I didn't want to have fun, and I even heard myself say "I don't like to dance." Well, that's a total lie. I love to dance. But fat me hated the way it made her body tired and her feet hurt.

I had been a failure on every diet before, because I never changed the way I thought and felt about food. I viewed each diet as a temporary thing. I was bailing out my boat every few years, but never fixing the leak, and the leak kept getting worse.

This time I knew I had to *change*. I had hit bottom. I wanted to *live*.

I found Medifast, a meal replacement diet, and I knew it was the right one for me. I was challenged by the wonderful veterans of the plan to just try the plan as written and see if maybe someone else was smarter than I was about how to be a thin person. Seeing as I'd never done it on my own, that sounded like pretty good advice to me.

I followed that plan slavishly for a long time. I lost the weight. With minor up and down maintenance struggles, I've kept it off.

My life is totally different. My body feels fantastic. I have tons of energy to move, play, dance, garden—whatever I want to do. I look great in my size six clothes. I can wear heels all day and dress up and feel pretty. I painted the outside of my own house, including extension ladder work.

If you haven't tried being thin, I highly recommend it. It's a fantastic experience. I'm here to tell you not only how to get there, but how to handle the radical life changes so you can stay there. You won't regret it, I promise.

II. BEFORE YOU START

Losing weight is hard. Being overweight is hard. Choose your hard.

Are You Really Ready?

Being fat sucks. But so does dieting. In fact, it's kind of a toss-up which sucks more. If you think about it, I'd go so far as to say evidence suggests dieting sucks worse than being fat, because almost every person who says they want to lose weight stays fat.

Dieting is about foregoing temporary pleasure in favor of long-term rewards. That sucks. Dieting is about deprivation, doing without comfort, entertainment, companionship, getting drunk off your ass, and chili nacho cheese fries. Did I mention it sucks? It sucks.

Being fat is also horrid. The physical aggravations, the shame, being invisible, being scorned, feeling alone and unlovable. The painful feet and knees. Making excuses to avoid finding out you have reached the point you have to buy two airline seats, or that the safety bar won't close around your gut on the roller coaster. The plus size department at the store, where they keep the vividly colored sacks of ugly. Being tired all the time.

I don't recommend dieting. What a miserable waste of effort. Most people are going to fail, and even if they do succeed, for most people it's temporary and they're right back up over where they started, ready to repeat the whole cycle again as soon as this episode of Seinfeld is over.

Before you slit your wrists in despair, what do I recommend? A lifestyle change. A radical change in your thinking and actions. A total shift in the direction of your life, that will take you down a new road full of long-forgotten or never-experienced pleasures. A change in your mind that leads to a joyful and healthy body.

This can be yours.

When you're ready.

Are you ready now? It's up to you to decide whether you've reached the magic moment. For me, I had to smack my fat ass on bottom with a resounding, public, *thud* before I was ready to change my life. I had to get so fat that climbing some stairs while traveling so exhausted me I sat down at the top and cried. Twice. My back in spasm, my feet in $500 custom orthopedic inserts, my hip joints and knees screaming, out of breath and humiliated. My lovely vacation in Mexico was a horrible experience because I was too damn fat to climb 150 stairs without crying.

That was my moment. I don't know if you've had your moment yet. If you haven't, you know what I think you should do? Take a minute to write down the things you don't like about being fat. Then fold the list up, put it away, and go eat whatever you want for a while. Stop doing whatever self-loathing diet/cheat/diet/guilt/binge cycle you've been locked in. Give yourself permission to relax. You might eat a lot of veggies. You might eat your way through all the appetizer sampler platters and dessert carts in town. It doesn't matter. If you're not ready to change your life for good, stop doing a half-assed job of it. Rest. Breathe. Eat. Learn to love yourself. Wait for your moment.

What if you're there? What if you've had it with being fat? What if you know your life must change now or you'll die before your time and make your pallbearers deeply unhappy?

Then change. It will be hard. So what? Being fat is hard too. Choose your hard.

Why Do You Hate Being Fat?

There are a lot of reasons to hate being fat, but it's important to be crystal-clear about what yours are. You need to make a list. It's your own, personal, custom-tailored inventory of misery. If you're obese, you have a list. Get *honest* and write it down.

And no, I don't care how "fat positive" you are. Being obese carries with it physical, lifestyle, and social tolls that are unavoidable no matter how supportive your community is of your freedom of expression or natural body type (or whatever they want to call condoning your overeating). Get honest, and write it down.

Here's my list I wrote five days before I started my new eating plan:

A Fearless and Searching Moral
Inventory of Just How Fat I Am

- 235 pounds
- Size 24
- Winded after climbing a flight of stairs, huffing a bit after two

- Right knee hurts some and crackles frighteningly
- Lower back hurts all the time
- Shoulders hurt, hips hurt, thighs hurt
- Thighs won't close without effort, which I can't sustain for long, much less cross my legs
- Back fat rolls
- Belly protrudes several inches past boobs
- There's a fat pad in the hollow of my throat
- I avoid things that involve walking, standing, dancing—I heard myself say "I don't like dancing" the other day. That blows.
- I avoid getting dressed up and going out—very little wardrobe, not that into swathing myself in a muumuu
- I don't feel sexy at all
- I'm avoiding social gatherings
- I will look like a gay pride float in the bridesmaid's dress
- I'm starting to have anxiety about being told to purchase two seats on the plane
- I'm tired. All. The. Time.
- I'm stuck in the vicious cycle of "too fat to want to go out and work off any of the fat, so I sit at home on the sofa eating to entertain myself, and figuring tomorrow I'll change."
- Can't wear my pretty pretty shoes.

I think it's interesting what things weren't on the list. My acne, which disappeared once I cleaned up my eating. The colds I would get, and my nighttime cough, both of which disappeared once I improved my diet and lost some weight. My orthopedic inserts, which I only needed because I was so fat I was destroying my own skeleton under my weight. It came to me later, as an epiphany, that the custom footwear was because of fatness, and not because of some mysterious weak arch thing that just happened to me. My denial was many layers deep, and full awareness took a long time.

My thighs rubbing together and chafing I simply forgot to write down. That painful rash really sucks. I had a special silicone roll-on for thigh chafing. Seriously.

It's hard to realize just how crippling obesity is, because it sneaks up on you. You think you're choosing the handicapped stalls in the bathroom because you like them better, and not because you have actually become handicapped and no longer fit comfortably in a normal bathroom stall.

Post your list somewhere you can check on it from time to time. This road will get painful. You will be close to giving up. Remembering the experiences you never want to have again can help keep your mind focused on the reason for your present suffering. You have to remind your greedy little subconscious that the pain of not having that Twinkie is substantially less than the pain of all the experiences on your misery list.

You're Not Healthy, You're Just Not Sick Yet

A fat woman's doctor said this to her recently. Apparently it infuriated her. Well, why not? Many of us fat people have normal blood pressure or cholesterol, even if it's just inside the line. We're not diabetic or on medications. Who is the doctor to say we're not healthy?

We're not healthy. We're just not sick yet. Obesity is life-threatening, and it will get you sooner rather than later. Think about all the really old people you know or see pictures of on their hundredth birthdays. Any of them fat? Bueller?

No. The fat ones die younger than that. We wear out our pumps and valves and such. We wear out the piping. We blow something out, like an overfull inner tube, whether it's in our brain or heart. We develop diabetes and are too fat to keep a close eye on our feet, and that goes south really quickly and in such a sad way.

I'm not going to throw a bunch of statistics at you. You know obesity kills, and you know you're not well. Just compare your energy levels to when you were thinner, or to your more slender friends. Think of the things that are twinging already, the nagging suspicions that all is not right beneath the surface of your skin.

If the iceberg has already crashed into your boat, in the form of blood-pressure or cholesterol meds, adult-onset diabetes, or back/joint troubles, well, it's time to get in the life boat and paddle off to a different metaphor. If you're not sure if you're sick, try making a list of every little physical ailment or aggravation. You will be shocked later to discover how much of your list vanishes when you lose weight. Even seemingly unrelated things like getting colds every winter or needing a lot of sleep.

Being truly healthy is the most wonderful feeling in the world. Give yourself that gift.

What Do You Want from Being Thin?

If you're going to radically change your mindset and life from that of an obese person to that of a thin person, you're going to need some positive motivation. It can't be all stick, right? We need some carrot.

What does your carrot look like? What's your vision for being thin? What experiences will that bring you?

When I wrote my list, before I started, I did a pretty lame job. The list of what I hated about being fat was very detailed and specific. The list of what I wanted out of being thinner was vague and general. Reading it now, it gives the impression I didn't really believe I would get there, and I wasn't at all clear what it would be like. I had been fat for a very long time.

If I were writing the list now, it would go on for ten pages. I have so many things, large and small, that rock my world about being at a healthy weight. And you will discover your own as you step through this journey.

My Motivation List:

- Bottom springs! [like Tigger—bouncy because his bottom is made out of springs.]
- Dancing moving playing fun to move the body
- Feeling sexy
- Looking good in clothes
- Looking good out of clothes!
- More energy for work, school, fun with friends
- More active social life
- Healthy body, strong, happy joints and heart
- Attention!
- Enjoying everything more, because my body feels better.

That's all I could come up with. I'm sure you can do better. Think back to when you were thin, if you ever were, or thinner. What experiences could you have then? How did your body feel? What things do you see your slender friends doing that you wish you could join them in? Where do you want to go, what do you want to do, who do you want to be?

Get it all on paper. Use it when things get tough. There is a vision inside you of the person you could be—call it forth and then make it happen.

Before Pics and Measurements

I know, I know, you hate the camera. You hate fat you, and you hate that shock of seeing just how fat you are in photos. Photos are the enemy of denial. When I got really big, somehow I convinced myself that I just kept taking bad pictures. No, honey, you did not suddenly become unphotogenic. You became fat enough that even compassionate fat-positive self-love couldn't make you enjoy looking at yourself.

If you're like me, you've been untagging yourself on Facebook and trying to be the one behind the camera when the group shot is being taken. There may be little or no documentary evidence of your current bulk. Well, later, you're going to want it.

Trust me on this. Later, when you've lost 30 pounds, you won't realize what a difference it makes. You'll be partway along, slogging in the trenches. You see yourself every day, as do the people closest to you. Gradual change doesn't get noticed the way sudden change does. But you can take a new picture and compare it to the old one. Yowza—you really did something.

And when you get to goal, how are you going to post that awesome side-by-side shot of yourself fat and yourself thin? How can you properly brag if you don't have the proof?

Do a photo shoot. There is someone in your life who can take pics of you as you are. Call it Step One of the life change: Getting Real. Believe me, your friends and loved ones have not failed to notice that you're fat. It's really not going to shock them that you are going to lose some weight. Take the photos.

Take front, back, and side views. Take your measurements and write them down. It's going to be very cool later to be able to say "I lost 18 inches off my waist." You want stats.

You have the fat—you might as well get yourself the bragging rights for when you lose it.

Keep a Pair of Fat Pants

You know the pair. This is the pair of pants you wear on "bloated" days. They're the one pair of pants that actually fit you. Mine were a size 24, and I wore them when I needed to feel "comfortable." What that means is that I was totally in denial about what a stuffed sausage I was in my 22s, and sometimes I just couldn't handle the squish.

Anyway, I had one pair of 24s. They fit perfectly. I kept them. I adore the photo of me standing inside one leg of them.

As you purge the old you from your life and your closet, keep the biggest pair of pants. Heck, keep an entire outfit. You will want it later.

III. WHERE DO I START?

The most important day of your new life is the day you accept that you didn't get obese because you knew what was best for your body.

Why Are You Fat?

In order to lose weight and keep it off, you're going to need to know why you're fat. Imagine you're hooked on pain pills. You decide you want to get off the pills. You stop taking them, the pain starts to come back, and you sit there, gripping the edge of your chair with white knuckles, moaning because of the pain, unable to function or enjoy your life.

How long are you going to last?

Do you think this scenario might have a better outcome if you look around, realize you have been taking the pain pills because of the hammer that's hitting you in the head every five minutes, and *stop the hammer*?

You need to stop the hammer. Otherwise, you're just trying to push an impossibly large boulder up a hill every day. Eventually you get worn out, slip and fall, and the boulder pushes you face-down into a plate of Twinkies and you regain all the weight.

Some introspection and the right application of effort can avoid this. I'll discuss this in more detail later, but for right now, let's start with the big picture. What kind of fat person are you?

Are you an emotional eater? A compulsive overeater? A stress eater? A bored eater? A partier who can't say no when others are indulging? Addicted to junk food? A "foodie" who just can't get enough of things that begin life with a roux? Trying to hide from men/attention/abuse? Someone who hates dealing with food and so eats too much once or twice a day, and your body is in starvation mode all the time?

If you were fat because of a legitimate medical issue, you wouldn't be reading this book. You'd be following your doctor's plan and getting your weight back on track. So let's don't waste another second of your life pretending you're just big-boned or have a slow metabolism. If you didn't have some sort of a problem with food, *you wouldn't be fat.*

Normal people, when they gain a few pounds, *eat less.* They take those pounds right back off. Their pants fit, all the time. We are not normal people. When our pants stop fitting, we squish into them, and then buy stretchy pants.

What is it about food for you? What makes it more important than health, mobility, an active social life, a longer lifespan, and being able to see your own junk? You need to know this. I'm not saying you have to have all the answers before you start, but you'd best start now on identifying the hammer and figuring out how to get it to stop hitting you in the head.

Pick the Right Plan for You

Different plans address different problems. If you're a junk food junkie, South Beach might be great, because it forces you to cook a bunch of fresh foods. If you're a carb addict, Atkins would force you to let that go for a while. If you're too busy to prepare food, a meal replacement plan could be your friend. If you're any sort of an emotional/stress/compulsive/bored eater, Medifast is great because everything is limited, even celery—there is nothing whatsoever that you're allowed to binge on.

There are countless diets available. I got lucky when I chose Medifast. My selection process went like this: I've done South Beach and loved it, but I'm too busy to cook that much. What else is out there? Oh, I have a friend who's lost about a hundred pounds, ask her what she did. Medifast? Oh look, packets! Neat. Sign me up.

I did not know at the time what it would force me to learn about myself. I didn't realize how the structure and strictness of it would change me. As an emotional eater, I ate to feel full. When I was very full, I would feel calm and safe. Guess what? My food plan did not allow me to eat a large pile of anything. Everything was weighed, measured, counted, and limited. This pushed me to a greater awareness of how often I abused food, and forced me to develop other coping skills.

Thank God.

So what are your weaknesses? How have you failed before?

- Do you like to "game" things, fiddle the diet around so you can still eat a plate of brownies? Maybe a points system is not right for you.
- Do you skip meals, get too hungry, and then overeat? Maybe you need something structured that requires many small meals each day.

- Do you pretend you're on plan when you aren't, and fall off the wagon when you're on your own? Maybe you need something with weekly in-person weigh-ins and meetings to keep you accountable.
- Are your taste buds over-excited and requiring massive fat/sugar/salt doses? Maybe a meal-replacement plan would let you calm them down.
- Are you a compulsive overeater? Maybe a 12-step program would be a good place to start.

There is no one diet that's going to work for everyone. Think about what you need to learn, and pick a plan that will teach you that. If you get partway in and discover you're failing, reassess. Did you pick the wrong plan? Or are you ducking the hard lessons the plan you're on is trying to teach you?

Know Thy Enemy—Understand the Science of the Plan You're On

All weight loss plans are not created equal. All of them that get any popular traction *work*, at least for some people who go on them. But why do they work?

Low carb plans get ketosis working for you. When you keep your daily carbs below a certain level, you enter a fat-burning state that speeds the process along. If you're on a low-carb diet, eating a lovely "healthy" piece of fruit can throw you off for 3 days, but eating some bacon would barely cause a blip. Carbs are the enemy.

Calorie-restricted plans work a little differently. The basic equation is: when (calories in) < (calories burned), you lose weight. Calories are the enemy. But you have to stay within certain parameters. I could eat 900 calories a day on Medifast because it was nutritionally enhanced and kept me in ketosis. But if someone ate a different 900 calories a day, it would shut their metabolism down into starvation mode and they wouldn't lose weight at all. There's a calorie and nutrition threshold you have to stay above on a straight calorie-restricted plan.

There used to be more diets where fat was the main enemy. However, that's a great way to lose your gall bladder. The body needs a certain amount of fat to have your organs function properly, and healthy fats help break down bad fats.

I'm not saying you should be planning to cheat on your diet. But you need to know how it works, in order to be able to work with it. You might find yourself having to choose the lesser evils from a work buffet, or being stuck at Disneyland a day longer than planned. You'll need to know what things you can fiddle with and what things are hard limits.

Do the research about the diet you're planning to use. Make sure it's one designed by doctors and nutritionists. Understand why they made the choices they made. Talk to people who've been successful on that diet and find out what worked for them. Talk to people who failed on that diet and learn why.

You're choosing *health*, after all. In order to choose health, you need to be armed with the right information for making healthy choices.

Eating Like You're On Your Way to the Electric Chair

You've picked a plan. You've got a start date in mind. Now what?

Do you eat like you're on your way to the electric chair? I certainly did. BRING IT. I had a lovely two week binge while my first shipment of food was on its way to me. I ransacked my mind for any stray cravings I could satisfy. I ate my favorite horrible foods, as often as I wanted.

Is this a smart thing? Maybe, maybe not. Some people are mature adults when they are about to start a diet. They start gradually reducing their carb and junk food intake. They get all fresh and springtimey in their hearts and colons. These are the kind of people who I want to stab in the eye with a fork, but bless their hearts.

Bless your heart if you're that kind of person. Acting in line with where you want to end up—that's wonderful. You won't hit the wall of carb withdrawal like all your fat friends are jumping up and down on top of you. Your transition to your new food plan will be accompanied by the soundtrack and field of flowers from a douche commercial. No lie.

Well, I'm not that kind of girl. I missed one thing in my binge. A certain fast-food chain had released a certain limited-time sandwich that involved fried chicken as the bread, and bacon and melted cheese inside it. I didn't get around to trying one before I started my diet. I craved it for months. Literally, months. It represented every delicious fried thing I could not eat, and it broke my heart. I still wish I'd tried it, back when I was a person who ate that sort of thing.

Now? Now I tried a tater-tot and it was so gross I spit it back out onto my plate. Fried food is not delicious anymore. That doesn't suck for keeping my weight off. But for the process of getting to where I could accept that I may never eat more than a bite of fried food again—for that process, it actually did help me to have my last hurrah.

Many of us fatties have a "you're not the boss of me!" mentality. We have to actively manage our spoiled brat selves in order to make more adult choices. For me, I avoided saying "I will never eat that again." Instead, I went with "I choose not to eat that today." When just getting started, it helped to remember that only a few short days/weeks ago, I ate _____. Over time, it became less important.

If you need a bender before you start, have one.

Cleaning Out the Sludge

When an alcoholic quits drinking in the movies, there's always a scene where they pour out all the bottles. Guess what? It's time to pour out all the bottles.

You have a food plan. Certain foods are on it. Most of the crap in your kitchen is not. Start at one end and move to the other. Throw out the things you can't give away, pack up the ones you can. Get them out of your house, *now*.

I had a bunch of perfectly good grains and beans that were not on my diet. They went in a box with a bunch of their off-plan friends. I gave that box to a friend and said, "No matter what happens, tell me they grew up and flew away to find great homes." I don't like to waste food, and so I needed her to throw things out for me. Yes, it's a weakness. But I recognized it and asked for that help from a friend.

What if you don't live alone? Well, tell your spouse and children they need to go live in a hotel until you reach goal. Okay, you probably can't do that. But you are going to need to clear out the things you can't handle having around. There will be some negotiation, and some petulance on the part of those not on a diet with you. Tough luck.

There is no reason in the universe that anyone must have junk food in their home at all times. If you and your spouse both love Cheesy Poofs, you may need to insist that Cheesy Poofs be consumed outside the home, or only enter the home in single-serving sizes that are consumed immediately by your spouse in another room. If you love Sugar-Frosted Cocoa Bombs and can't stand Frosted Wonder Cakes, then it doesn't matter how many Frosted Wonder Cakes are in the house because you don't want to eat them. Steer your spouse towards their indulgences that are not on your weaknesses list.

You are not punishing your children if you don't have junk food in the house. This is not child abuse or torture. In fact, you're giving them the gift of being able to learn more healthy eating habits. Don't apologize. There's nothing to apologize for. Just start feeding everyone better food, and refuse to buy crap at the store. They'll catch up soon enough.

As you start dropping the weight, you can distract your spouse from the lack of junk with more vigorous and enthusiastic sex, and you can distract your children with more active outings. Everyone wins.

IV. LOSING—THE PHYSICAL PROCESS

I'm hungry. So what? I'm always hungry. This is no longer news, or a problem.

Screw Exercise When You're Obese

Do you know how hard your body is working all the time, just being fat? Sitting still you're working hard enough to put yourself in an early grave. Deciding it's time to lose weight and starting some Boot Camp to do it? Suicidal.

They say that every extra pound you weigh puts four extra pounds of strain on your knees. All that fat is impacting your heart, lungs, muscles, joints, and bones. Talk to fat people about their feet. Hear any stories of plantar fasciitis, orthopedic inserts, fallen arches, walking fractures, and just general pain? Have any of these yourself?

You've been living your life at some baseline activity level. For some, this is the sofa and a scooter to get around at the grocery store. For some, it's a minimally active life, parking close to your destination, wearing comfortable shoes, and avoiding events that involve a lot of standing. For some, it's 75-minute step classes three times a week and mountain biking on the weekends.

It doesn't matter what your baseline activity level is—just leave it alone when you start your diet. Change your eating habits. Don't put the extra pressure on yourself of changing your activity levels at the same time.

If calories in < calories burned, you will probably lose weight. There are some medical conditions, and some combinations of the wrong calories (or too few) that will not support weight loss. But if you pick a medically sound food plan and stick to it, your chances of success are high.

With exercise alone, your chances of success are *not* high. Let me share some math to prove it (hang in here, this is worth it). Let's say you want to use exercise to take off some weight. You only burn 100 calories a mile, whether you're walking or running. You've probably been eating more than 100 extra calories a day, so you're going to need diet changes at a minimum to limit your intake to what you burn in a day. Then you add in walking a mile every day. A pound of fat represents 3500 calories. That means it will take you 35 days of walking a mile, after you reduce your intake to break-even, to lose your first pound of fat. Wow. At that pace, Gandhi would have a hard time staying motivated.

Let the diet do the heavy lifting at first. For me, I weighed 235 pounds. That's a *lot* on a 5' 2" woman. My knees, hips, back, etc. were already feeling the strain. I decided that I didn't want to ruin my knees any further by pushing myself to work out. I felt like crap, I was living on 900 calories a day, and exercise could wait.

This had the benefit of making it possible for me to stick to my diet. If I were pushing myself to feel even worse, I would have given up. I believe that making one big change at a time is enough to focus on.

This strategy had the benefit of letting my body direct my movement. As I got lighter, I started feeling like moving around more. I found myself puttering around my house instead of sitting on the sofa. My bathroom got cleaner, my laundry got folded and put away all the time. I started walking more, most noticeably while shopping. For hours. Wandering around, trying cute outfits on my new smaller body. I started wearing shoes with small heels instead of my industrial ugly ones—heels give your thighs a workout all day long.

Eventually, I started shaking my booty at various dance clubs. I anticipate having some sort of a regular exercise program at some point. It's a healthy thing to do, and I absolutely approve of strength training for women, as well as cardio for overall health. You will have less sag in your skin if there's more muscle for it to hang onto. You should exercise, definitely. But do you need to start exercising to lose weight? No. Should you start exercising when your body is already under siege? No.

Take one thing at a time. Let your body lead the way.

Kill Your Taste Buds—Eating Clean

The American diet is a disaster, right? Fast food, take-out, frozen dinners, processed processed processed. Many people feel they're virtuously eating healthy when they eat a microwaved frozen vegetable that comes in its own "cheese" sauce.

This is not healthy and you know it. MSG, artificial flavors, salt, fat, sugar, corn syrup, artificial sweeteners—they've all done a number on your taste buds. Your taste buds are desensitized, overwhelmed, and overstimulated. It's like a porn addiction—the longer you sit in your basement watching porn and avoiding human beings, the more hardcore and intense of stimulation you need, and the less attractive the kind, wholesome girl with a crush on you becomes. Plain steamed broccoli has a crush on you, and you're ignoring her.

Junk food is a gateway drug. To more junk food.

What to do about it? Eat clean. Shop the perimeter of the grocery store. Seek out fresh, simple foods, and then don't doctor them up. If you're on a meal replacement plan, eat the meals more or less as they are provided, without trying to turn them into a Cadbury Creme Egg.

Your food will seem bland and boring for a while. It might be hard to make yourself eat a salad that doesn't get 95% of its calories from the blue cheese dressing you have ladled onto it. But try. Know that your taste buds will readjust, faster than you think.

I often eat my salads without dressing. I eat cabbage plain, with just a little salt sprinkled on it. I order my meat in restaurants without any sauce, butter, or oil on it. Plain steamed food tastes wonderful to me.

Did I start off there? Hell no. I was putting enough butter on my food that I could buy it at Costco. I live alone. I was quite happy to go through a drive through a couple times a week. I ate canned chili with cream cheese in it, scooped up with tortilla chips. I was a fatty with fatty taste buds.

I went through withdrawal from the overstimulation. It went along with the withdrawal from being able to comfort eat, and the physical carb withdrawal. It was all incredibly painful and I just suffered through it.

But now I'm a girl who spits out a tater tot. It was disgusting. I can't imagine going back to blue cheese salad dressing—all that fat, for what? Yuck. The veggies are delicious. Now my taste buds are my allies in my lifetime task of keeping my weight off.

A fat man commented on the protein bar I was eating—he said they all tasted chalky to him. Yes, they do, when you're comparing them to deep-fried calamari and tiramisu. But when you're comparing them to plain grilled chicken breast with a little salt and garlic powder on it, they taste like rich deliciousness.

Reset your baseline for how food should taste. It will help your health long-term, and it will help you stay on your food plan now.

Yes, You Have to Give Up That One Thing

There's always a thing. It might be one, it might be several, it might be a whole large category like "sugar." But there are things that you can't handle. They're creamy deliciousness, melty goodness, or sweet temptation. Whatever they are, they are just too damn good.

Some of them are going to be allowed on the diet plan you're on. Some of them are going to be encouraged on the diet plan you're on. Does that mean you should eat them? No.

Certain foods lead us to want more of them, or just more period. If a food makes us want *"more more more"* it's a trigger food. Our trigger foods can change over time. I didn't think I had any actual triggers when I started my diet. I wasn't aware of anything prompting a binge of the "dozen donuts then hide the container" kind. But then again, I never tried to deny myself anything. If I wanted a dozen donuts I'd eat them over the course of six days, but I'd still get that dozen donuts in my body.

When I started my diet, I did have enough self-awareness to know that I was not capable of handling melted cheese. The Medifast plan would have allowed me up to eight ounces of melted cheese in a day, as long as it was a reduced fat cheese and I was on an allowed modified plan. In fact, someone posted about how she ate a cup and a half of roasted peppers and four ounces of melted cheese as her dinner on PMS days. Did that sound amazing? Yes. Was it a little too amazing? Oh yeah.

I didn't want to risk it. I feared I would want more cheesy goodness, more fried food, more more more. I went like four or five months without melting cheese. I'd have the occasional string cheese stick, but I wouldn't heat it up. After a while, my taste buds had cleared out and I felt more confident about my commitment to the plan. I put some cheese in frittatas, melted a little on top of things. But I watched myself closely: I measured to the gram, and never ever rounded up. I knew I was not to be trusted, and I was ready to yank my new cheese privileges away at the first sign of greed, cravings, or rationalization.

You might know what some of your triggers are. You might know that an open jar of peanut butter is not safe with you in the house. You might know that you can never stop at one brownie or piece of cake. You might know that a pound of bacon is always one serving for you. Whatever it is, let it go. Take it off your list of allowed foods. I don't care if it's "healthy." It's not healthy for *you*.

As you discover new triggers, take them off your list of foods too. There is no point to making this process any harder than it needs to be. You're fighting on enough fronts without bringing your kryptonite into it.

Two months into transitioning into more "normal" foods, I went to see my doc about a runny nose and weird itchy places. He thinks they are an allergic reaction to something I'm eating. He recommended an elimination diet to find out exactly what I'm reacting to. When he handed me the week one list of foods, he looked concerned that I would freak out about how restrictive it is. I scanned it, saw that it had protein sources and veggies on it, and said, "oh sure, no problem." Then he showed me the uber-strict three-day regime after week one, where you can just have lamb, a few veggies, and a couple carby things, and I said, "well, lamb isn't my favorite but for three days no sweat."

I have learned some serious non-attachment to my food. As long as he wasn't going to make me eat carbs I didn't care how short a list of foods it was. I'll eat lamb + broccoli for three days. What do I care?

I remember suffering with Candida for years longer than I had to because I wasn't willing to give up wheat, sugar, and potatoes forever, and a whole lot more for the cleanse phase. Those days are gone. No food is worth feeling like crap, or even a little off. No food is worth staying fat for.

Give up your darlings. You'll be glad you did.

Handling Cravings

Cravings are the powerful urges we get to eat off-plan foods. They can be tightly laser-focused on one thing, and we walk around like zombies with our arms out, saying "Pizza… pizza… pizza…" They can be broader, and we just have an itchy "sweet tooth" or "snackish… crunchy…" feeling.

However your cravings show up, they're a problem you need to actively address. Luckily there are lots of things you can do. Any of them are just ideas. If something doesn't work, or doesn't keep working, try something else. Experiment until you find the best way to manage yourself given your relationship with food.

Cravings Management Strategies:

- Ignore them until they go away. This is a "don't feed the beast" strategy. Whatever you give energy and attention to increases. Whatever you ignore will eventually give up and go sulk in a corner. Quietly. Which is just how you like that pesky entitled brat who is screaming for Twinkies.

- Distraction. If you're busy doing something else, it's much harder to fixate on that food you're not eating. Get out of the house, do some gardening, whiten your teeth (ever try to eat with those trays in your mouth?), take a sleeping pill and go to bed, exercise, whatever. Do something that has nothing to do with food.

- Diagnose the problem. What has prompted this craving? Did you have too many carbs earlier in the day and now you're extra hungry? Did you forget to eat your last meal yesterday and now your body is freaking out because it doesn't have enough fuel? Are you failing to get a minimum amount of fat/salt/potassium/etc in your diet and your body is trying to get its nutritional needs met? Look over your food log. Ask people who are doing the same diet you are. Do an internet search for "salt cravings" or whatever and see if there might an underlying nutritional lack you can correct.

- Dig into your feelings. Is there something else going on that's triggering you to want this food? Did you just visit your mother and now you want an entire pie? Is work extra stressful? Did you just have a fight with your partner? Are you bored or lonely? Evaluate how you're feeling. Dig deeper. The more you know about the root causes of your individual desire to eat, the better-equipped you are to control yourself.

- Snack. So you can't have bacon right now. Would a dill pickle give you something to put in your mouth and at least handle the desire for salt? Different plans will have different allowed snack foods. Try sugar-free Jello or popsicles, diet soda, pickles, celery sticks, a couple ounces of lean protein, a cheese stick, etc.

- Drink water. It's harder to want to eat if you've just poured a quart of water into your stomach.

- Pray. Whether you're on a formal 12-step program or not, turning it over to a higher power can help many people.

- Use a mantra. Mine was "That food is not for me." I found it surprisingly powerful, especially when confronted with samples in the grocery store or a buffet table. *That food is not for me.* It would calm me right down, reminding me that I did not choose to eat that food, even though it was available to me.

- Huffing. I huff a lot of food. Carbs and sugar smell amazing to me. I have discovered that smelling them can be satisfying all by itself. I can have an enjoyable experience of the food without polluting my body with it. In fact, I've lost the taste for sugar and carbs make me feel like crap, so smelling them has actually become the only way I enjoy these foods. Try smelling deeply of the food that's making you crazy and see if that doesn't alleviate the craving.

- Imagine eating the food. Scientists recently did a study where they had people repeatedly imagine eating a food. The people who imagined eating thirty bites of the food ate less of it than those who imagined just a few bites, and they both ate less than people who spent no time at all imagining eating that food. Your mind is powerful, and a vivid mental experience of eating a desired food might remove the urge to do it physically.

- Think dirty thoughts. Picture the "dirty man hands" that were in that bowl of candy before you came along. Get a very clear picture in your mind of how often people fail to wash their hands after using the bathroom. Imagine those dirty hands combing through the buffet food, preparing it in the kitchen, etc. Know that anyone could have sneezed or coughed on it, and there could be clumps of snot and spit on that apparently delicious item right now. Still want to eat it? I thought not.

Play around. Come up with your own favorite strategies to handle cravings. They do not have to get the better of you if you don't let them.

Handling Restaurants Like an Entitled Princess

"OMG what am I going to order at this restaurant there's nothing on plan on their menu??!"

We can try to avoid restaurants, or only go to restaurants of our choosing, but eventually we will fail. There will be a work function, or fat relatives in from out of town who reject your healthy eateries, or a first date who picks the restaurant and you don't want to act like a freak about food. What do you do then?

Don't panic. Bring a towel.

Just kidding about the towel. But don't panic. The mental shift you need to make is this: a menu is *never* a list of dishes to choose from. It is always a *list of ingredients* they have in their kitchen.

Say you're low-carbing it and you want to get a salad. You carefully peruse the salad list, and find one that seems close. Then you have to ask the waitperson what else is on it. This is that interviewing process that makes you look freakishly high-maintenance. You end up telling them "no croutons, salad dressing on the side, no beets, grilled chicken instead of fried" and five other modifications. Then what comes out of the kitchen will have honey-coated walnuts, parmesan cheese, and carrot shavings all over it, none of which you were expecting, plus the croutons will still be on it. Do you send it back? Fussy bitch. Do you eat it? Cheater. Do you spend ten minutes moving the high-carb carrots off to the side of the plate? Way to impress the boss, food freak.

It's so much better to just tell them what you want. If you want a salad, read over the available salads to see what veggies they have in the kitchen. Then put together your own salad: "I want a salad of spring greens, tomatoes, cucumbers, and hearts of palm. No dressing." Guess what? You order it that way, you will get exactly what you want, every time. They can't really bitch about it because you're asking for cheap ingredients they have in the kitchen, and they're going to charge you the same they would if they had to cover it in feta and bacon-wrapped foie gras.

My most common dinner order is a steak (not a fatty cut of meat like rib-eye, something lean), grilled, "no butter no oil no sauce dry spices okay, no sides," and veggies like broccoli or green beans "steamed, no butter no oil no sauce." The steak could be chicken breast or fish, as long as it's grilled, baked, or steamed, and not battered, breaded, or fried. The veggies could be any veggies that the restaurant has in their kitchen, or it could be a salad. To select the veggies I might scan the menu to see what they have, but I don't put too much stock in what the menu says. I usually have the best luck ordering my meat and then saying "and what can you steam for me?" They quickly suggest broccolini or whatever they have about, and it's a very short conversation.

By ordering exactly what I want and starting from the ground up, I avoid all the unexpected "treats" like a pile of mashed potatoes on my plate or cheese as a garnish. I skip the dinner rolls or whatever other surprises might come out with my food. Best of all, no interrogating the waitperson about what else comes with the food that isn't listed on the menu. We skip that entire conversation.

If anyone comments on my order, I can easily explain that I prefer the taste of simple foods. It doesn't have to be a thing. The actual time with the server can be short, reducing the amount of time you feel exposed as a fatty making a fuss about food in front of other people.

Bear in mind that you can become a skinny person. Then you'd be ordering like this all the time, and it would just be how you eat. Many skinny people don't put a bunch of crap on their food. Waitpeople do not seem the slightest bit surprised or unsure how to handle it when I order simple grilled/steamed food. I have never gotten the slightest bit of resistance or push-back about how I should try it with the sauce. Start eating like a skinny person now, and these habits will serve you in good stead long-term.

Not Eating Around Busybodies and Food Pushers

Restaurants are easy. Your hostess's five-course meal, the pizza party at work, the drinks at the bar, or the cupcakes one of the other moms made for a class party—these are hard. Each of them comes with food pushers, saboteurs, invested givers, and busybodies. These people are a problem, no doubt about it.

Somehow, these people have decided that it is their business what you put in your mouth. They've come to the conclusion that you're rejecting *them* if you reject their food. They think you're the enemy of fun if you don't drink with them.

Well, honestly, they may be right. You might indeed be the enemy of fun. You are making changes. You are rejecting an entire lifestyle that revolves around conspicuous consumption. You are choosing to no longer be a person who helplessly displays, through the rolls of fat on their body, the power food and drink have over them. By making this choice, you are forcing them to confront their own choices.

Some of these people are just hateful or jealous. Don't be surprised if your thin friends start bringing you takeout or an entire pie. It upsets the natural order of things when their fat friend starts looking better. If this continues, it could get out of control. Their fat friend could start looking *better than they do*.

What are these people going to do? They're going to push food on you. "Just try a bite." "I made it just for you." "One small piece won't hurt." "You have to eat normal food again someday, right?" "Come on, just have a drink! It's no fun if you don't." "Aren't you hungry? Aren't you going to eat anything?"

First of all, it is your body. You wouldn't let someone push you into having sex you don't want to have, so don't let them push you into eating food you don't want. You need to police the boundaries of your body. "No" is a complete answer.

However, it's not always a polite answer. You can certainly play around with snappy comebacks if you want, but I tend to prefer a mannered deflection. Tell people you just ate and are still full, you don't feel well and don't want to become ill, or you have gum in your mouth and the mint won't go with _____, etc. One woman tells people she has food allergies. It's true, after all—food makes her swell up like a balloon!

You can avoid having to say anything at all by strategic use of props. If you're at a cocktail party, get sparkling water with lime in a pretty glass. It will look like a cocktail and no one will wonder about it. Plus, you'll have something in your hands, and that will help keep you away from those Costco mini quiches on the food table. At a restaurant, order some tea to "settle your stomach." If you know they will not be okay with you refusing birthday cake for a coworker, accept a piece and say you're taking it back to your office for later.

Bury it in a trash can. Distract, deflect, avoid, and you can skip most of the nonsense.

I do not want to suggest you *get* a new eating disorder, but you can learn from your friends with eating disorders. They are very comfortable with the words "I'm not hungry." Or, they cut their food up into small bites and shove it around on the plate without eating it. In an episode of Skins, the anorexic girl makes it through an entire meal without anyone knowing she never ate a bite, by loading up a fork and waving it around as she talked. People saw her about to eat and didn't notice the food never made it to her mouth. If the event only has fatty carby sauce-laden disasters of food, it's much healthier to eat before and after. Sometimes discretion is the better part of valor. Confronting the busybodies just takes so much *effort*.

If all else fails, get back in their face. "Why does it matter to you what I eat?" See if they can come back from that and keep pressuring you.

Is it reasonable you have to go through all this to keep people off your back about what you eat? No. But your life-change is stressful enough. If opting out of these conversations makes it even a tiny bit easier, it's worth it.

Take Your Vitamins

You're restricting your intake of food. Some essential nutrients will be shortchanged. You need to look at your particular diet and the nutritional composition, and decide what enhancements should be made.

Check with your doctor to help you design your plan and double-check your decisions.

Vitamins To Consider:

- Multivitamin: this may or may not be a good idea. On a meal replacement plan, the space food includes 100% of the RDA of the essentials, and a multivitamin can cause toxicity. On a simple calorie-restricted plan, you might end up deficient in some things, and a regular supplement could be a good idea.
- Omega 3s: your body needs these good fats for a whole slew of things like heart health, and it needs them more when dieting, to control hunger and help with fat burning. Good fats help break down bad fats. Take flax seed oil, fish oil, or the like. It will also help keep you regular.
- Fiber: some plans may not provide enough fiber. Supplement with psyllium or another fiber supplement. Watch out for extra sugar, carbs, or artificial flavors—you can get plain psyllium in capsule form.
- Biotin: any rapid weight loss can cause your body to decide certain things aren't essential. Like hair and fingernails—eek! Biotin helps keep this to a minimum.
- Probiotics: acidophilus and bifidus are the healthy critters that live in your gut. They assist digestion and help keep the evil critters under control. Yes, this is the official scientific language for this process.

There may be other things you should consider. Talk to the people who have been doing the diet you're on for a while. The "vets" of a plan can be a treasure trove of information. Again, check with your doctor about your overall plan.

Don't Take Weight-Loss Pills or Get Surgery

Yes, you're fat. Yes, you want to stop being fat *right now now now are we there yet???*

Well, tough. You did not gain all that weight in a day, and you're not going to take it off overnight either.

This is a *good thing*.

You need the time on your new food plan to learn a new way of living. You need to be forced to confront the reasons why you overeat. Otherwise, you're just stopping the pain pills while the hammer still whacks you in the head. Taking the slow road lets you find and stop the hammer.

No matter what method you use to lose weight, you must find and stop the hammer if you're going to keep it off. You must learn why you overate. You must learn new coping skills to deal with the things that pushed you to food. You must unplug whatever is driving the cycle of eating more calories than you burn.

This learning can't be skipped. Taking a magic pill that suppresses your appetite or prevents your body from using the fat you eat—what happens when you stop taking it? Are you going to stay on that pill for the rest of your life? You really think that's healthy? Side-effects from appetite-suppressing drugs include psychotic episodes, depression, and suicidal thoughts. Yay—sign me up!

What about surgery? Sure, people lose a crap ton of weight the first year. Then most of them start gaining it all right back. There was a man who got the surgery and lost a bunch of weight, but would order fried chicken jumbo buckets for the office. He would set out the food for everyone else, and then drink the quart of gravy himself. One woman post-surgery gets her salad with blue cheese dressing on it plus extra on the side to dip into. Another one chews her food and spits the bulky parts back out. She sucks off the fat and salt and ejects anything that would take up room in her smaller stomach. She will get an extra plate for this at a restaurant. Can you imagine? A plate of chewed cud?

They still eat like fat people. They still think like fat people. They do everything they can to circumvent the good things from the surgery. And the weight comes back and they die like fat people—if the side effects of the "cure" don't kill them first.

Surgery and pills do not cure Fat Person Brain. They do not solve the underlying problem. You do yourself no favors trying to find a shortcut. The only road to a thin and healthy body is through changing your relationship with food.

Can you do that? Yes. Will you? I don't know. But you most certainly will not by wishing for a miracle drug. Instead, believe in yourself. Get some therapy. Pick a plan that gives you time to learn about yourself. Turn it over to God.

No matter what you choose, you have to do the work one way or another. Why destroy your body with medical interventions with pathetic long-term success rates when you have to learn new eating habits anyway? It's just a delaying tactic. You can do better, *now*.

Do Take Drugs When You Need To

My first week on my new food plan was one of the most horrible experiences of my life. Carb withdrawal can be a nightmare of fatigue, headaches, crabbiness, hunger, cravings, and misery. Doing without comfort eating is the shock of being a toddler and having your bankie taken away. Knowing you *can't have more* induces primal panic.

It blows.

No need to make it any harder than it has to be. I took sleeping pills five of the first seven nights on my diet. I would lie there obsessing about what I couldn't eat, when I could eat next, what that food would be, how hungry I was, whether I should go eat something, etc. Inside my brain, it was like one of those heroin withdrawal scenes in the movies. Not so much with the sweating and the shakes, but inside? Oh yes. I was a total junkie mess.

I drugged myself to get through it. Am I proud that I needed to do that? No, I think I'm pretty darned pathetic, actually. Am I proud that I made it through? Hell yes. The pills were a small part of my arsenal, and they let me get past the worst bit. Soon enough I learned that hunger is not a crisis and that going to bed hungry didn't do me any damage. After that I learned to enjoy the feeling. But that all took time. Some strategic pharmaceutical intervention helped buy me that time.

You know what drugs you need. Anti-anxiety meds, anti-depressants, sleeping pills, whatever. Now is not the time to go off your medication. Now is a good time to use whatever supportive tools you need to assist your main focus: getting the weight off for good.

Work with your doctor to shore up your weak spots. One thing at a time. Right now it's reducing your weight. Get all the help you can.

Drink Your Water

Lots of it. All the time. Drink at least 64 ounces of water as a bare minimum. Better yet, drink at least half your body weight in ounces every day. A 200 pound person should drink at least 100 ounces of water.

I'm not going to get into the full scientific explanation for it, but you need it for weight loss. Water is an essential component of the chemical process that breaks down fat for fuel. If you shortchange your body on water, you can be doing everything else right and still fail to lose weight.

Diet soda and Crystal Light do not count, either. Get pure, clean water moving through your body, and it will help you. It will flush out fat. It will also flush out the toxins and hormones you're being flooded with. Fat cells store toxins and hormones. When they break down for fuel, their nasty passengers are dumped back into your body and have to be purged.

What if you hate water? Consider it a growth opportunity. You are no longer allowed to hate vegetables, either. Grow up and figure it out.

Try a special glass, or using bendy straws. Try it iced, fridge-cold, room temp, or hot. Try making yourself drink 16 ounces before every meal, or after every meal. Try tap, bottled, fizzy, flat, or flavored with a lemon slice. Keep experimenting until you find a combination that is tolerable. Over time, you'll probably come to love it, if you give it a chance.

Drink your water.

Yes, You Must Log Everything

If you bite it, write it. Everything that goes into your mouth must end up in your food log. The food plan you choose may come with a tracker app for your phone or online. Or use one of the many general purpose ones available.

There are three times when you must log your food: when you are starting the diet, when you find you're getting sloppy/not losing, and when you transition at goal: off the weight loss phase to maintaining your losses.

When starting the diet or when getting sloppy, it's a powerful tool for accountability. You need to be able to see what you ate. You need to see the numbers: calories, carbs, fat—whatever the critical measurements are for the plan you've chosen. When transitioning, you need to know what's going in, so you can adjust things if you start gaining again. You must have accurate data in order to make effective course-corrections.

If you don't log, you will lie to yourself.

You will convince yourself that those couple bites don't matter. Well, on some diets a couple bites could have enough carbs to kick you out of the fat-burning state. A couple bites could easily lead to more bites if not reined in. You will underestimate the amount of foods you eat, if you don't weigh/measure them and log them accurately.

When I eat my favorite flax seed crackers, I open a bag and divide it into 14 gram servings. One-half an ounce. By the time I eat 14 grams and drink a glass of water, I feel satisfied. But if I sat there with the bag open, I am quite sure I'd eat five times that without a second thought. When I cook, I weigh every ingredient before it goes in the pan.

Is this a bit obsessive? Sure. Does it work to keep me honest? Yes. Does it let me see my intake of calories and carbs and compare it to what the scale says and how my pants fit? Absolutely.

Log your food. There's an app for that.

V. LOSING—THE MENTAL GAME

Cheating is not a success strategy.

It's Not a Diet, It's a Lifestyle Change

A diet is okay when you're one of those horrible people who want to take off five pounds so their adorable little girl six-pack really *pops*. A diet is a great idea when you want to take off fifteen pounds of beer fat so you can wear your wedding dress in a size four instead of eight. A diet is the perfect thing when your inclusion in the Mission to Mars is contingent on your weighing a stone less than you do.

But a diet is not okay for losing a large amount of weight and keeping it off.

A diet is inherently about tension and deprivation. A diet brings to mind living off of grapefruit and a single lettuce leaf. It makes us think of plain celery sticks, and quite frankly, if you get excited about plain celery sticks you're going to need to rethink things. Maybe some therapy. You're not doing this "fat" thing right at all.

Anyway, a diet is about doing without until you go off the diet. That creates tension. There's a tension between today's suffering and tomorrow's joy. You're just waiting until you lose the weight, because then you can eat like a normal person again. Hooray!

No. Not hooray. First off, let's look at some normal people. Have you seen the obesity statistics lately? Been inside a superstore and looked at the customers? Gone to the county fair? We are fat fat fat around here. "Normal" involves batter, frying, HFCS, batter-dipped and fried HFCS, giant portions, rich sauces, preservatives, and enough salt to replace what a fat girl cries into her pillow at night. When I go out to dinner and watch what people consider to be "normal" it revolts me now. I can't believe they eat all that. Yuck.

Eating "normally" means being fat. Please take a minute and absorb that. Eating like our dominant culture eats means being fat like most of the people you see on a daily basis. One more time:

Eating "normally" means being fat *forever*.

You may get closer to thin for a while, on your latest diet. Your friends will politely tell you that you look great, and the more honest among them will actually say things like "You know you're going to gain it all back again." And then you will gain it all back again, and more. Because the pattern is to yo-yo steadily upward, and unless you make some serious changes, you're not escaping the pattern. You haven't yet, right?

How do we escape the pattern? We make a lifestyle change instead of going on a diet. Instead of thinking "In six months I can have this double-stuffed cheese-dipped chocolate-smeared goodness" you think "That is a disgusting mess that will kill me, and I choose not to put it in my body." We embrace the idea that we are changing our relationship with food forever. We let go of the tension of deprivation, and welcome the rich goodness of simple foods.

Your taste buds can change. You can get to where simple, nutritious foods taste amazing to you. You can learn to like new vegetables. You can become a person who eats like a thin person.

The first step is letting go of "temporary." Replace it with "this is how I eat." If you're a petulant defiant brat like me, replace it with "this is how I choose to eat today." But move it into the present. Own it. Be the change you want to see in the world.

(Sorry about that. Couldn't help myself.)

Create a new normal for yourself that hearkens back to an earlier time. Your new normal can be whole nutritious foods without a lot of embellishments. You can tell people you eat Paleo or you're on a health kick or you fear cancer—or tell them nothing at all. The crap we put in our bodies now is an invention of the last sixty years. Healthy food was a fad for a lot longer than that. You can never go wrong with a classic.

Small Goals, One Day at a Time, Rewards

You need to lose fifty or a hundred or three hundred pounds.
Wow.
That's a really big number. That's a horrifying number. That's an *impossible* number.

Make it less intimidating. Break it down into smaller pieces, and lure yourself along to one small achievement at a time.

Many people find that having smaller goals lets them set their sights on something that seems achievable. It's not a hundred pounds, it's ten pounds ten times. And then it's not even ten pounds ten times, it's *this* ten pounds. Just ten pounds, looking no further than that. They set their tickers to reflect a ten pound goal and call it "Goal #2." They manage themselves so they don't freak out about the giant task ahead.

What do you need to manage yourself? For me, I needed to set a more "realistic" goal. I felt like 150 was a number I could envision. When getting started, I had 150 on my ticker and "we'll see how it goes and maybe I'll stop at 170 if I like it there" in my mind. It was only much later, when I realized success was attainable, that I decided I didn't need to settle for 150 just because I had gotten up to 235. I ended up losing down to 135 before I felt I had the body I wanted to live in for a long time.

Some people focus on one day at a time in order to not get overwhelmed. Telling themselves that they're making a change forever can provoke a defiant opposition, or trigger feelings of helplessness. Instead, saying "just for today I choose not to eat ___" can make it manageable.

Many people find rewards are helpful for reaching mini-goals. A charm for a charm bracelet for each ten pounds lost. Mani-pedis, massages, cruises, a new dog, designer jeans, etc.—a series of things to work towards. Just make sure to never use a food as a reward. It's not about getting to goal so you can eat the forbidden again. We're making a permanent lifestyle change, not delaying all the good things for once we're skinny. All rewards need to be not food-related.

I found I didn't need to buy rewards, because I was so pleasantly distracted by the intrinsic rewards that the weight loss brought me. I had so much more energy, attention, cute clothes, etc., that I didn't need anything else. Or maybe more accurately, I was so busy rewarding myself with new shiny things and experiences all the time that I didn't need "extra" rewards for attaining goals. My favorite reward of all is people telling me how hot I look, and you can't buy that. You have to work for it.

Do some reflection on yourself and what you need to keep your head in the game when confronting a large task. Then actively manage your mind to keep you on track.

Commitment, Not Will Power

Will power is hard. Will power is pushing a boulder made of lard up a hill, until your mental muscles give out and the lard explodes all over your ass again. Will power is no good for a lifestyle change.

Commitment is much better. If you're committed, it's just what you *do*. You get up in the morning and you eat like you eat, because that's the only option. You don't eat like you think you should only on days when you can muster the strength to force yourself.

If you find yourself in tension with your food plan, ask yourself if you're trying to push a boulder up a hill. Reflect on what you want out of this. Do you want to be able to play with your grandkids? Have awesome sex? Rock some size eight designer jeans? Get off your blood pressure and cholesterol meds?

Whatever it is, be clear about your vision for your future. Know that you can have that future if you choose to.

Commit to that future. Commit to yourself. Take all the choices and *moods* out of it. Do you always feel like going to work, brushing your teeth, being nice to your mother? No. Do you do it anyway because you made a commitment to your employer or yourself? Yes.

The New York Times ran an amazing article by John Tierney about decision fatigue. It discusses our ability to resist temptation and make choices that are better in the long run rather than feeding immediate gratification urges. Apparently our will power is in short supply, which is not a shocker. What might be more surprising is that it's depleted not just by resisting temptation, but also by making any sort of decision. Later in the day, after we've made a lot of choices, we are less able to resist temptation and stick to our diets because we have decision fatigue.

The cure for this is simple: take choice out of it. You have a plan, you have a schedule, and you stick to it no matter what. You're not forcing yourself to do anything, or making choices all day long about what to eat. You're just in a groove, on your plan, losing weight.

If You Were as Smart as You Think, You Wouldn't Be Fat

It's time to admit the truth: *you don't know what's best for your body.* Listening to your body has led you down a garden path paved with gluttony and weight gain. Your "inner voice" is the voice of a greedy entitled brat who will do *anything* to get her way.

Listening to your mind has been a mistake too. Your mind says you know better. That you are capable of figuring out what your body needs. That you know best, so you need to "tweak" the rules of any diet to make it work for your special needs.

Are you fat? Then you don't know better.

41

Early on in my journey to lose a hundred pounds, someone wiser than I am challenged me. She suggested that perhaps I don't know better than the doctors at Johns Hopkins how to lose weight (they designed the Medifast program). That struck home. Those doctors, or whichever doctor you choose to listen to, have the benefit of years of training and study, as well as hundreds of clinical trial participants. They have tested out their theories prior to publication and actually know what will work to get the fat off my ass.

So I followed their plan. I had great success on Medifast, and before that on South Beach and other diets. There are many great plans put together by doctors and nutritionists. These plans have proven success rates. It doesn't matter which one you choose, as long as you pick one that will force you to learn and change, and teach you healthier eating habits. But once you pick a plan, stop tweaking.

A little tweak here, a tiny adjustment there, and next thing you know you've convinced yourself you just have a fast metabolism and so you need to eat 6 tablespoons of peanut butter before bed. No. You don't. You need to follow a plan and learn something new.

You suck at making it up. Stop doing it, *now*.

Just One Bite—Destruction Testing

"One bite won't hurt." Well maybe, maybe not. The problem is, you can't know if it will hurt until it has already hurt you.

You're on your plan, you're through the worst of the withdrawal, and you've lost some weight. You're starting to feel like you've got your legs under you again and you can do this. Then there's that food. That delicious food. One bite—what could that matter? It's hardly worth putting in your food log it's so insignificant. You eat it, and it's delicious.

What happens after that? For a small percentage of people, you say "yay, that was good, now back to my food plan." I won't say there aren't people who can handle one bite like it didn't matter at all. But are you one of them?

What if you're not? What if instead you're one of the majority of people, for whom one bite can shatter their serenity? Now that you've had a bite, you're back in the world of choices. You've thrust yourself out of commitment and back into will power, pushing that boulder up a hill. With every moment of the day, every time you're around food, you have to ask yourself, "Should I have some? How much? One bite? One small piece?"

The rationalizations are constant: "One bite didn't hurt before, I still lost two pounds that week." "It's my birthday." "I'll hurt her feelings if I don't try it." "I can handle it, I can stop anytime."

Will you? Will you stop anytime? You can't know for sure until you try it. For most people, a bite is the first step to a binge or a slide. Once you've let yourself know you can cheat, you've strengthened the greedy inner brat. You've fed the beast, and the beast is now stronger. Can you shove it back in its cage and lock it down? Maybe.

Maybe is the problem. Maybe you will, maybe you won't. Most people won't, and then they're off the diet, getting fatter again, and working up the will power to restart in a month, a year, a decade, or never. Why engage in destruction testing if you don't have to? The only way to find out if it's going to derail you is to get derailed.

It's a useless, pointless, self-destructive experiment. If one bite of food is so important, perhaps that's what you should be looking at instead. Why is one bite so important I'm willing to risk my health and my future hotness? What does this bite of food represent? What feelings am I trying to feed?

Stay on your plan. Give it everything. So what if you're a little obsessive about it? You're yanking the pendulum hard to the side of sobriety, and yes, later you will let it swing back to the middle and find whatever degree of moderation works for you long-term. But now, in the weight loss phase?

Strict. No bites, licks, or tastes (BLTs). Following a plan 100% works. Half-assing it never works. Will 95% work for you? Maybe. Maybe not. Don't risk it.

The Science of Figuring Yourself Out

Roasted salted nuts have a trigger effect on me. It's the classic "one is too many and a thousand isn't enough" problem. I can't try one and be satisfied. If I have one, I will obsess about them until I binge and realize that I have no control over nuts *at all*.

Carbohydrates have a physical effect on me. After eating too many carbs at once, it's no longer a matter of will power or what's on my food plan. My body has some sort of blood sugar meltdown. I eat more carbs for a while, and then I switch to protein. I eat lots of protein, trying to get my blood sugar restabilized. No matter what I eat later, after I have that big dose of carbs the rest of the day is shot. It's a different feeling from craving a particular food, or being triggered by one food. It's a physical thing that happens with my metabolism, especially when I've been low-carbing it.

These are things I have learned through long trial and error about me, about my metabolism. What do you already know about you? What things send you off your game?

The important thing for you is that you avoid the shame spiral when you've eaten off your food plan. You didn't do anything wrong or bad. You're not weak. You're doing science about what works for your body and what doesn't. Take a step back when you've eaten off your food plan, and ask a lot of questions:

- Why did you eat it?
- Was it emotional, mental, or physical hunger?
- What feelings were you having when you made the decision to eat it?
- What happened in your body?
- What did you then eat later?
- Was the problem the particular food item, type of food, or quantity?
- At what points could you have made different choices?
- How can you make a plan for the future to make different choices?

The other day I was short on sleep and out running errands. Being short on sleep makes me hungrier and reduces my stores of will power. It was getting close to time to eat again and I didn't have another healthy meal with me to start into, so there was a lack of planning in play. I was feeling virtuous because I'd gotten up early to do something unpleasant, so I had a mental sense of entitlement. And then I started having the thoughts about "Why can't I have a bag of Ruffles like a normal person? I'll get a small bag. It's a snack food, not crack cocaine."

I got the bag of Ruffles. 400 calories, and 38 grams of carbs. The carbs were the problem. After that I ate several protein bars, seeking their 24 grams of carbs each. Later in the day I ate more eggs and cheese than are in my normal food plan. I ended up eating about 1200 calories more than I had planned to overall. It wasn't just that bag of chips.

The analysis is important. I know I am vulnerable when tired. I know that there's a spoiled brat inside me who needs to be reminded that I'm not a normal person, and there are physical things which happen when I have even a small bag of Ruffles. 2 Ruffles—fine. One Goldfish—no problem. A bag? Forget it. I had gotten a little lax with my advance planning and should have had another meal with me.

These are the things I can control to avoid going off plan in the future. Try to get enough sleep, even if that vampire novel is very suspenseful. Have food with me. Squash the brat.

What are the things you can control to avoid going off your plan?

Perfectionism—All or Nothing

Many of us fat people are perfectionists. Somewhere along the line we decided that if we can't do something perfectly there's no point in trying to do it at all. We bring this line of thinking into our diets, and use it to let any small misstep derail us utterly.

What if you have a bite of a food that's not on your plan? Or you end up out longer than you thought, stuck somewhere without access to your on-plan food, and you have to choose the least of available evils? Or you set a goal of 20 pounds lost by June first and you've only lost 18? You've gone off your plan. Now what do you do?

Many of us immediately say "I'm already off my diet. This is my *chance.*" Presumably the idea is that on some mythical tomorrow we'll be perfect enough to do it perfectly, but in the meantime, since we've already failed, we should take advantage and eat everything in sight.

We tell ourselves there's no point if we can't do it perfectly.

We've already failed.

But have you really? You've taken a small step off-plan, or reality has failed to give you the results you wanted on your timeline. But that's not actually failure. That's one small action.

Once you've blown it the calories don't become free, either. It's not a binary thing—on plan or off plan, with no difference in consequences. Off plan can be small, or it can spiral into huge. The

45

question is not whether you fell off the edge of the cliff, but how soon can you get out your ice axe and self-arrest?

Don't throw out babies with bathwater. You don't have to scrap your entire future every time there is a small setback. Watch yourself for all-or-nothing thinking.

When you've strayed, the time to stop it is now. Not later, not after eating the rest of the bag, not after hitting a drive-through to take advantage of your off-diet window of opportunity. Get back on plan and move forward from here.

When the Scale is not Your Friend—Immediate Gratification

"I want what I want and I want it *now*!!!!!"

This is the rallying cry of our inner brats. They are loud, demanding, powerful creatures. They are also wily, manipulative little bastards. Our inner spoiled brats have us wrapped up tight around their little fingers, dancing to the tune of their temper tantrums. "Dance, monkey, dance! And while you're up, get me a pizza."

Recognizing the brat is a bit easier when she's demanding junk food. It's a challenge round to see her in action when she's stomping her little feet for some more carrots. It's the final bonus round to see her coming at you over the scale.

"It's not working." "It's not fast enough." "At this rate, we'll never be wearing a size four for the cruise." "What's the point if it's going to be this slow?" And then she starts in with how you need to eat a pizza to "jump-start your metabolism" and you're sunk.

Your body is going to lose weight at its own pace. If you have carefully chosen a doctor-recommended weight loss plan and have been following it slavishly, you *will* lose weight. You will not lose three pounds a week every week. You will not be able to see a drop on the scale every day. It will take time.

It will also go up and down. Weight normally fluctuates up and down several pounds during the day, and a couple pounds from one morning to the next. You weighing more today than yesterday could be because you exercised (tiny muscle tears hang onto water as part of their repair process), you're constipated, you didn't drink enough water, you are retaining water because of some hormonal thing, you had more salt than usual, or the moon is full in the seventh house of who freaking knows?

One thing I can tell you—a pound of fat is comprised of 3500 calories of fuel. If you've been on your plan, then you did not eat 7000 extra calories yesterday and gain two pounds of fat overnight. We know it's not that.

This is a good time to take the long view. It took time to get fat. A lot of time and dedication, really. Consistent hard work. It's going to take a long time to get thin again.

But you know what? That's a good thing. Use the time on your diet as a learning process. Study yourself. Get inside your mental, emotional, and physical reactions to food. Get therapy. Talk to people. Notice how you are with food. Learn everything you can, and change.

You can't change overnight. If you magicked off the weight with a twinkle of your nose, you'd still have the same relationship with food and eating habits. You'd go right back to piling on the weight. Welcome to the world of yo-yo dieting.

The time it takes to lose the weight is a gift. It's a time-out from acting out your unhealthy relationship with food. Use that time-out to shift the relationship, build skills, and form a plan. Don't expect things to change instantly.

Where would you rather be a year from now? Pouting because that diet you stayed on for six weeks didn't make you skinny? Or proud of yourself because you stuck with it for six months or a year and accomplished something amazing?

Even slow losers get to goal.

Methadone is a Bad Idea

Unless you're one of those rare people with a health issue that makes them gain weight no matter what they eat, if you're fat it's because you have a problem with food. You may have a compulsive eating disorder, be a foodie, get too busy and not eat often enough, not take time to cook and eat too much processed food, stress-eat, comfort-eat, eat when you're bored, drink too much beer, eat too many white foods, have sexual traumas that make you want to hide from male attention behind a wall of fat, have a killer sweet tooth, or all of the above.

Whatever your reasons are, you have a problem with food.

One more time: there is a *problem*. With *food*.

Believe me, I hate admitting this as much as you do, maybe more. I still cringe away from the words "binge" or "addiction." There is a part of me that is convinced my weight gain just happened to me sort of by accident and that nobody really noticed I was fat. If I just pretend it never happened, then I can pretend I don't have a problem with food.

Well, I do, and so do you. Figuring out the exact flavor of your problem with food is one of your exciting challenges right now. Yay!

Lots of things can help you on your journey to lose the weight and figure out why you had it so you can keep it off. Foods that mimic your heroin are not one of those helpful things.

The diet I chose was Medifast, a meal replacement plan. You eat a lot of space food from packets. The meals include things like brownies, puffs, crunch bars, etc. What if you're a person who likes to demolish a tray of brownies at a sitting? What happens if you eat the space food brownies?

For some people, nothing. For more people, they manage to eat only as many replacement-brownies as they're allowed for a while, and then they lose it. They eat too many of them. Also, they keep telling themselves it's okay to eat brownies, and that they *have to have* brownies, and so they're more likely to eat the real thing again when the diet is over.

People lose their minds trying to come up with a way to mimic their favorite thing. They pile on fat-free whipped topping, PB2, sugar-free syrups, and low-fat cream cheese until they've concocted a horror-show of chemicals that no one should ever eat. It's all in an effort to stimulate their taste buds the way they used to be stimulated by that food. That heroin food you just can't resist.

What a great message to send yourself, right? Even when you're on your diet, exercising tight control over what you take into your body, you still are helpless to avoid that one thing. You have to make the methadone version of it. You have to.

Really? Do you really have to? What if you just don't? What if you just walk away from brownies, Cadbury Creme Eggs, or cream sauces? I didn't let myself melt cheese for the first maybe five months on my diet. Melty goodness was over my line for deliciousness. I didn't need the temptation.

Guess what I learned? I learned I didn't need it after all. I learned I can live without it. I learned I can let the crispy cheese bits on the edge of someone's plate go back to the kitchen untouched by my hands.

That knowledge is something I will have forever. Would I have learned that if I'd worked melty goodness low-fat cheese into my daily meals? No.

I'm not saying you should avoid all food that tastes good. But learn where the line is. Are you just trying to stimulate your taste buds like your favorite addictive foods did? Then skip it. Eat something simple and nutritious. Let your taste buds calm down and your body learn some wisdom.

Ritual

Ritual is a powerful thing. It can be your ally in this journey. Anything you do over and over gains strength from repetition.

My favorite diet ritual was my pickles and cream cheese nightcap. The plan I was on allowed for up to two tablespoons of cream cheese a day, depending on what else I ate. Your body needs a certain amount of healthy fat, to keep your gall bladder working properly. Cream cheese was my favorite delivery method.

Every night, I'd have two dill pickle spears and two tablespoons of cream cheese. I'd lick the cream cheese out of the tablespoon. It was always the last thing I ate before bed.

This ritual became a safe refuge because I did it over and over. If I was out late, and out of food for the day, I somehow knew I'd be okay because I'd get to have pickles and cream cheese before bed. Once I had eaten this, I knew I was done eating for the day, because that was always the last thing. It helped me avoid late-night snacking because I never ate anything after the pickles and cream cheese.

There were other rituals that helped me. I always drank at least a pint of water after eating. That helped me feel full. I ate every two and a half hours all day long, at the same exact times. That way I always knew I just had to make it to my next mealtime and I'd get to eat again. I always had a large meal for lunch. I logged everything I ate.

They say it takes 21 days to form a new habit. Do some thinking about what rituals might help you stick to your diet. Then practice them until they become a habit. Let the power of ritual and repetition assist you towards your goals.

You may have had rituals that worked against you. If there was an overeating routine you had, whether it be Friday night drinks and nachos or a private calming moment with a pint of Häagen-Dazs, it's no longer serving you. Find a way to step out of that routine and break its habitual power over you. It will take time, but it's worth doing.

The power of habits is why so many people drastically change their social life when they quit drinking or smoking. It's hard to keep being in the same environment with the same people and not keep doing the same things you've always done. Give yourself permission to make whatever changes you need to make to step out of your unhealthy rituals and into your new healthy ones.

Your Self-Sabotage Routine

Do not trust your brain. It will lie to you.

Seriously. You got fat because you have a fat brain. It is full of ideas that support you overeating, eating the wrong foods, and staying fat. It all works together—fat brain, fat eating, fat body.

Going on a diet isn't enough to stop the cycle, because your fat brain wants to drag you back to the status quo. It wants the status quo with such power that I believe fatness is harder to kick than heroin—both kill you, and yet we see a whole lot more fat people than junkies. This is *hard work*.

Here are the kinds of things fat brain likes to say:

- Just one bite won't hurt
- I've already gone off plan, now is my chance
- I need to practice eating normal food
- I've been so good I deserve a "treat"
- I can't let people know I'm on a diet
- Nobody's perfect
- I'm only human
- I'll do what I want and you can't stop me!
- I can't waste food
- I need to kick start my metabolism

Don't go down without a fight! The benefit of a strict diet plan is that you can easily see when you're off plan or wanting to go off plan. Then you can carefully inspect the inside of your brain and see what nonsense it's been trying to feed you (pun intended). Fight these ideas. Root them out. They are no longer serving you.

One bite will hurt. One bite of a food not on your plan opens up a Pandora's box of temptation and decisions. Now you have to ask about every freakin' thing that crosses your path—"Do I eat this? How much? One bite? A small piece? I didn't gain with last week's one bite, so obviously it doesn't matter." And away you go.

You need to practice eating normal food? Uh, no. No you don't. You've been practicing that your entire life. I practiced right up to 235 pounds. That's enough practice for a lifetime. I practiced, I got fat, now I need to learn something else.

The "treat" thinking is insidious. I was raised with food as a special treat. It's hard to stop myself from going down this mental road.

Who cares if people know you're on a diet? Believe me, it's no secret that you're fat. We wear that fact right there on the outside where everyone can see it. People are going to have their own judgments about what you eat, whether you're fat, thin, or anywhere in between. Let them have their judgments; it's none of your business. You focus on you and what you need to do for your health.

Nobody is perfect, and you are only human. Yes, it's true. But guess what? So is every person who performs an act of heroism, raises a child, or walks their dog every morning. Part of being human is having the ability to make choices. Those choices can include doing something well, consistently, and with honor. If you decide to follow your food plan 100%, it is easily within the realm of things that humans are capable of to live up to that. Don't insult humans that way—we're pretty remarkable creatures.

Yes, you can do what you want, eat what you want, and no, we can't stop you. Nor do we want to, really. It's all in your hands. Watch your inner spoiled brat for this oppositional thinking. Do you really want to be eating yourself to death now because someone told you that you couldn't have dessert 30 years ago?

Wasting food—this is another hard one for me. Right now there's some food in my fridge I shouldn't have bought in the first place, that I'm struggling over what to do with. It's a little too fatty for my usual food plan, and I don't like how I feel when I eat it. My mouth loves it, though, and my fat brain says it's wrong to throw it out. Well, my body is not a trash can. This is remarkably hard to remember.

Kick-starting your metabolism—this is a very popular rationalization for going off a diet when things aren't moving fast enough. We have problems with patience. The desire for immediate gratification over long-term happiness is what led us down the road to obesity to start with. If a diet slows or stalls for a couple weeks, we tell ourselves we need to shake things up by eating more food for a couple days. Uh, no. The proper reaction to a slow or stall is to get stricter on the diet, not throw it all to the winds.

Each of these ideas and so many more are easily addressed. You know everything you need to know to examine a "fat brain" thought and logically tear it to shreds. You just need to step back and do it.

Watch your lying brain. Catch it in the act. Don't let it keep you from the life you really want.

VI. LOSING—THE EMOTIONAL QUAGMIRE

It's not about what you're eating. It's about what's eating you.

It's Not a Sin, It's a Food Choice

Somewhere along the way we ended up with all this moral context around our food choices. A Ding Dong isn't just a stupidly sweet petroleum product we occasionally opt to eat. Instead, it's wickedly delicious, a sinful treat. What exactly is "sinful" about it?

It's not really "good" or "bad" to eat a certain food, right? It's just a food choice. Different foods have different effects on our bodies. If we look at our cars, some fuels are healthy for our engines, like gasoline, and some are not, like shampoo. It's smarter and creates less roadside drama when we run our cars on gasoline and avoid shampoo, but that doesn't make it "good."

We use language that gives eating choices moral content. This feeds into our feelings of guilt and shame about what we eat. If you've ever found yourself eating your way through a shame spiral, you know that being ashamed of something doesn't stop us from doing it. It's all part of the package to feel guilty about eating something, take it home to eat it in secret, and end up eating a whole lot of it to stuff down that feeling of shame.

As a negative shameful thing, calling it "bad" or a "sin" doesn't help us stop doing it. What about as a positive thing, as an enticement?

As long as certain food choices remain "sins," that makes them more attractive as well. It becomes a pleasurably guilty indulgence, a bit of naughtiness. In general, I enjoy a bit of naughtiness—that's not a disincentive to me! But if I can strip away the "minor sin" emotional overtones, perhaps I can view a bag of Ruffles as what it is—a bag of MSG-laden snack food that will momentarily excite my taste buds, then make me feel like crap and overeat the rest of the day. A poor fuel choice. Not a scrumptious bit of wickedness.

I can't see any way in which making food a sin helps us have the bodies we want. Let's take away some of its power, and just let it be fuel.

You Must Take Care of Yourself

May people wind up in bad places in their lives because they don't feel they should be taking time just for themselves. Somehow, they've come to believe that self-care is selfishness and should never be indulged in. They feel that the partner, kids, job, clients, whatever must always come first.

What would you tell an exhausted friend? Would you say, "You're right, honey. You should keep working yourself into an early grave so your kids don't have to lift a finger at home," or "Forget about sleep and eating healthy food, your clients need you to be on-call 24/7 for their manufactured crises"? Really? Because that's what you're telling yourself.

Logically, what happens if you consistently neglect self-care for years? Something breaks down. You fall apart: you become ill, have a nervous breakdown, or just drop dead in the harness. Is this going to do your kids or clients any good? Who's going to take care of them when your heart gives out?

You have to turn this fat thing around. You have to. For them, if you can't manage to admit it's okay to do it for you. You need to be alive to do anyone any good at all.

It takes time to prepare and eat healthy food. It takes time to exercise. It takes time to drink enough water and get enough sleep. You have to be refreshed enough to remember why it's worth the effort to resist temptation and eat right instead.

If the raging sense of guilt continues to be a problem for you, force yourself to make time for seeing a counselor. Work on this issue. Find the roots of your belief that domestic or professional martyrdom is a high calling. Turn it around.

No one gets to the end of their life and says, "I wish I'd spent more time at work." They say that they wish they'd followed their dreams and invested more in their relationships with loved ones. They wish they'd expressed their feelings more and allowed themselves to be happier. Guess what? Losing the weight can help you with all of these. You will have more energy to follow your dreams. You'll be in a better space for genuine quality time with loved ones, rather than being so fatigued all the time. You'll remember that you're worth standing up for, and that will lead to expressing yourself and being happier.

Make the time. If you can't act as though you believe you deserve it, get some help for this issue.

Self-care isn't selfish. It's self-love, the first building block in true love of others. Model self-love for those you care about, to teach them to love themselves as well.

Special Occasions—Make it About the Friends, Not the Food

Imagine it's your birthday, and you're having a party. Someone has brought a lovely cake. One of your friends is allergic to wheat and you know she won't be able to eat the cake. What do you do? Do you tell your friend to stay home because eating cake is the most important part of the day?

No. You most certainly do not. You tell your friend to come and eat what she can and celebrate the day with you. The cake is there as a pleasurable indulgence for those who choose to partake of it, not as a gauntlet that must be run by every person at the party to prove their love for you.

Remember this when you're on the other side. The not-eating side. You're at the event or special occasion for your friends or family members. You're there to celebrate life, love, friendship, achievement, etc. Even if the event is a wine tasting, you're not there for the wine. You're there for the company and the enjoyment that being a social monkey around other social monkeys brings us.

This can be hard to keep track of, when everyone seems to be raising a glass at once, or eating pizza together. But in any large group, if you look more closely, you will find that some people are not partaking in whatever it is. If it's alcohol, some people are designated drivers, some are sober, some don't like the taste, and some don't want the calories. If it's pizza, some are allergic to tomatoes or wheat, some are lactose intolerant, some are vegan, and some don't want the calories. Don't focus on the majority and feel excluded. Instead focus on what you are sharing in—the *fun*.

Other people will lose sight of this on occasion. The deflection strategies discussed above in the section on busybodies and food pushers will help. But you can also be more direct—"I'm here for my friends, not the food. I hope that's okay with you." It would take a lot of nerve for someone to reply that it wasn't okay.

Remember the upside. As they're all getting drunk and fatter, you get to watch them get stupid with a crystal-clear memory of everything they say and do. And tomorrow, you'll be fitting in smaller jeans while they'll be moaning about how they shouldn't have.

You get the exact same experience of love, companionship, and celebration, without the extra calories.

Yes, You Eat Like a Freak Now

One of the things that's hardest to come to terms with when changing your eating habits is how that makes you appear to others. Or at least, how we think that makes us appear to others.

From the inside of my head, when I would order something grilled with some steamed veggies, I felt like there was a giant neon sign above my head saying "oh yeah, sure, look at the fat girl being all high maintenance and demanding in a futile quest to not be hopelessly fat forever and ever hahahahahahaha…" I know, it's a lot to fit on a sign.

Would it have been better to order a deep-fried onion like other people at the table? To eat my seafood fried and covered in tartar sauce like a normal person? Would that somehow have kept the secret that I was fat?

Uh, no. Eating fatty food did not hide my fatness. It didn't even clearly communicate to the world my devil-may-care *joi de vivre*. It just quietly announced, to anyone who cared enough to notice, that I was a practicing overeater.

What really happens if you start eating healthier in public? Nothing much. A couple friends or family members will pout and push a little. Most people won't say anything at all. A couple people will join in, saying "You know, put my salad dressing on the side, too." Wait staff will just bring you steamed veggies with no fuss whatsoever. And a buffet table is not going to give a crap one way or another about whether you partake.

That doesn't mean it's not hard inside our own heads. We feel that neon sign blinking there in the air above us. For me, it helped to embrace that I now eat like a freak. I now and forever order like a fussy high-maintenance *skinny* person in restaurants. I scrape sauce off things. I don't eat fried food. So what? It's my body.

My skinny body, beyatches.

Handling the Sabotaging Partner

Your partner (or parents, housemates, siblings, children, friends) says they love you. Most of the time, you even believe those words when they come out of their mouth. But then you go on a diet.

You're working harder than you've ever worked on anything in your life. You're committed. You are making changes *happen*.

They bring home donuts and fried chicken.

You come home and your favorite junk foods are laid out to tempt you. Or they order a pizza to "celebrate your diet success." Really? To celebrate my staying on my diet you want to make we walk the plank into a giant tub of full-fat ice cream? Awww, thanks for thinking of me, I love you too!

Treats are delivered with an expectant smile, like you're supposed to thank them. Well, that's not going to happen.

When dealing with the sabotaging partner, it's important to remember two things: 1) they might just be a jerk, and 2) they might not be. Let's look at these possibilities in turn.

No relationship is perfect and we'd be lonely forever if we insisted on perfection. But some relationships are a lot less perfect than they need to be. I don't think I'm going to shock anyone by saying that very often people with a weight problem have an accompanying or underlying self-esteem problem.

Lack of self-esteem leads us to settle for much less than we deserve in the loving respect department. We either seek out partners who will treat us like crap right off the bat, or we encourage this behavior to increase slowly over time by allowing it. I am not blaming the victim here. What I am saying is that it does take two to tango—if you leave the dance floor entirely, they can't keep treating you like crap.

If your partner is leaving you "treats" because they're a jerk, why are they doing it? To keep you fat. To keep you hating yourself. That lets them keep you right where they want you, under their control. It also lets them keep feeling better than you, or at least no worse. If you keep failing at your diet, they hope you will believe yourself a failure. They are counting on the death of your dreams. And could you bring them another beer while you're up.

Only you can decide if your partner falls into the jerk category. If they are, then you're going to need to decide if they're unredeemable. Take a hard look at your relationship. Stretch your imagination. Can you see a future where the two of you are happy together? Can you picture them happy for you when you achieve personal or professional success? Can you imagine them proud of you?

If you can imagine these things, then get started creating them. Stop taking crap. Tell them you're done taking crap. Do it in a firm way, if that's the approach they need, or ask gently, or carefully negotiate. Let them know that things need to change between you. Identify the specific behaviors and words that make you feel disrespected and unloved. Get the help of a counselor. Remember that you helped create this situation, and it's going to take a lot of work from you as well as them to change it. You need to change yourself into a person who nips that crap in the bud, and that's a really hard thing to do while still inside the relationship.

If you can't imagine your partner treating you well in any universe, it's time to get out. Take whatever measures you need to be safe. Bury your dead and move on. Get started changing yourself into a person who nips that crap in the bud in her *next* relationship.

Let's look at the possibility that they're not just a jerk. If that's the case, why are they trying to tank your diet?

Maybe they're just oblivious. You've been together for 15 years, and for 14.99 of those years you really liked it when they brought home donuts and fried chicken. They could just be acting out of habit and trying to be nice to you.

If this is the case, you can try pointing out to them that things have changed, and you no longer want them to bring you food as a gift. Many times a clear statement of the new rules for presents will turn things around.

What if that doesn't work? What if they "forget" and keep doing it? Accept the treat, say "thank you," hold eye contact, and dump it in the trash in front of them. Seeing their "gift" get thrown away can be a more powerful behavior modifier than any conversation.

What about emotional reasons for trying to sabotage you? Two big ones are the fear of losing you, and not wanting your body to change.

They might be afraid you're going to leave them. A lot of people do end their relationships when they lose a bunch of weight, so it's a valid fear. Think through what getting skinny could mean for the two of you. Are you still going to find your partner sexy? What about lifestyle changes? Are you going to be happy with them if you get into biking or dancing and you have to do it alone because they're still on the couch you used to share? How are you going to handle all the new male attention? Is it going to turn your head and make you start shopping for an upgraded arm-accessory to go with your upgraded wardrobe?

If you want to stay with your partner, then you're going to need to get them on board with the idea of a changed you. Talk to them about their fears. Let them know how sexy you find them and that you are making these changes for you, not so you can leave them. Ask them to be your ally in creating your new life.

Don't try to push them to change with you. It's much better to lead by example, quietly, in a relationship. Change your diet, get more active, and see if they get inspired by your success. Whether they do or not, keep your mouth shut about what you think they ought to be doing. Just because you got a memo to radically change your life doesn't mean theirs is due to arrive at the same time. Instead, focus on maintaining your connection. Keep doing the things you enjoy together that don't revolve around food. Let them hear, see, and feel that you're not going anywhere.

There's another possible reason why someone who is not a jerk might be trying to sabotage your diet: they like you as you are. Personally, I am attracted to fat men. Not men with 10 extra in a pot belly, but men with 50 or 100 extra on top of strong muscles. Giant mountains of men just make me want to *climb* them. It's not the only body type I'm attracted to, but it's a recurring favorite.

What if fat you is your partner's physical ideal? Marilyn Monroe was not a thin woman, and she had men all over the world swooning. People are attracted to a wide range of body types, including fat ones.

Your partner sees a girl they swoon over. They get lucky and find out that the two of you are compatible in relationship. They get you into a relationship. Right now, the A-Team theme music is coming up and someone is saying "I love it when a plan comes together."

Then there's a screech of a needle on a record as you start non-consensually taking away the body that turns them on so much. Seriously. Did you ask them? Did you negotiate this? No. You're just changing the body they love.

I'm not saying you should ask them before starting a diet. Their attraction does not give them rights to make the decisions about what goes in your body or how you look. But you can be understanding of what you're asking of them. You can apologize, and let them know you hope they'll find the new you attractive as well. Most people have a range of body types/sizes they respond erotically to, so they might weather the transition just fine once they get over grieving the loss of the junk in your trunk.

You can try to sell the upside of the changes: greater flexibility and endurance, more energy, increased libido. That could help quite a lot.

But if it doesn't help, well, you might lose them. There are a few men who found me attractive at 235 who still find me attractive at 135. But by and large, fat Freya and skinny Freya appeal to different men. I was single through most of my weight-loss journey, so I didn't have to lose a partner as I lost my weight, but you might.

If you're about to lose your partner, make sure you're committed to changing your life through changing your body. If you know in your heart that you're going to go back to your old habits in a few months, well, maybe you could be on the board of directors of an orphanage right now instead of on a diet. There's got to be something productive you can do with your energy and drive to change something in the world.

If you're committed to radically changing your life and becoming a thin and healthy person, apologize to your partner and let them make their own choices. Be as loving and gracious as you can if they decide to go. While loving someone no matter what is a lovely ideal, the fact of the matter is that sex matters in relationships, and attraction matters in sex. Forgive them for being who they *always were*.

No matter what type of partner you have, or what their motivations are for sabotaging you, talking can never hurt. Keep asking them what they're feeling, what their fears and concerns are, and what they need from you.

And then dump those donuts in the trash and go for a nice long walk through the Juniors' department at the mall. In a few short months, you could be wearing clothes that cute. How's that for motivation?

Don't Feed Your Emotions

I really wish I had some magic answer for this one. Believe me, I do. In fact, right at this very moment I'm anxious about something and a snack would really hit the spot.

What does it mean to feed our emotions? For me, I'm a comfort eater. When I'm really full, I feel safe, like nothing can get to me inside my little cottony cushion of fullness. As a result, I eat when stressed, lonely, sad, or angry. I also eat when bored or in celebration. I'm not sure I have any emotions that I am not capable of eating to handle. When all you have is a hammer, everything looks like a nail.

Take a little self-inventory. Think about when you overeat. What are you feeling at the time? What happened before? How do you feel after? Something is better, right?

The problem is that it doesn't stay better. After the brief euphoria of the binge or the fullness, there's a quick or slow crash. The effect wears off. You may have a shame spiral. You may just go back to feeling mildly depressed and run down, weighed down by the fat you're carrying. No matter what your emotional situation with your eating and your weight, if you are eating to deal with emotional stuff you will never ever fix the emotional stuff that way.

Whatever loneliness, boredom, anxiety, anger, or sadness you had before you ate is still there. It's shoved down under a layer of carbs and fat, sure. But it's still there. Eventually you're going to have to deal with it.

As they say in AA, "If you aren't willing to be uncomfortable, you probably aren't willing to be sober." Not stuffing our emotions with food means we have to deal with those emotions.

Ugh. What a pain in the ass that is! It involves all this self-reflection and awareness, dredging stuff up, admitting that some things need to change in your life, dealing with the past, etc. It's an unpleasant task at best. If it were fun, you would have done it long ago, instead of trying to fix your problems with an upraised fork.

Well, it may be unpleasant, especially at first, but it's so worth doing. If you can identify the source of the feeling that sends you to a self-destructive coping mechanism, you can deal with the feeling and skip the self-destruction. You can tell someone "don't talk to me that way" and be thin, instead of taking it and staying fat. You can join a bridge club and make new friends and be thin, instead of sitting home lonely and fat. Your options are *unlimited*.

Dig into the feelings and you won't need to dig into sludge.

Mood Swings and Psychotic Bitchery

Oh yes. You will have it. You will have the crazy. Going on a diet is like coming off any drug. You have to force yourself to stay away from your favorite things. You are suddenly doing without your favorite coping mechanism for the ups and downs of life. Someone took your teddy bear and eviscerated it with a chainsaw in front of you.

You will have the crazy.

Moods will swing up, with a glorious manic edge to them. You're changing your life, you're in control for the first time in a long time, anything is possible. You have renewed energy from being in ketosis or having dropped some extra baggage. Life is your oyster.

Moods will swing down, or sideways, with alarming speed. Road rage is a serious concern. Coworkers will suddenly become the most annoying people on the planet in the history of ever. You'll see a commercial for fast food and literally cry because you can't have your old friend anymore. Memories of old painful events will drift up into consciousness to be dealt with. You'll snap at people.

You won't even mean to do it. It's just that you used to have a soft cushiony pillow of a coping mechanism, and you took it away. You're off balance. You need to learn a new way to live. Unfortunately, that takes time.

You can do the best you can to stay aware and not take it out on people. That's hard, and you won't be perfect. The best you can do is give people a heads-up. "I'm going through withdrawal from carbs and it's making me a little insane. If I am cranky your direction I apologize." And then try to notice when you actually do it, and apologize again.

There's nothing wrong with you. The mood swings are not a sign that you should eat carbs again. They're a sign that you're changing your life in drastic ways. Any emotional work you do is going to help. But some of it is just physical and hormonal, and you simply need to ride it out.

You'll stabilize again. It may take a few months or longer, but it will get better, I promise.

Just Get Some Therapy Already

Yeah, sure, there are some people who love to be in therapy. For them, there's nothing more wonderful than someone's undivided attention as they lovingly sift through the wreckage of the past, the delicate archeology of pain. I admit it—some years I am one of these people, too. Given unlimited funds, yes, I'd be in therapy until I puked.

But what if you're not? What if the idea of talking about your mother or your feelings makes you want to puke before you even walk through the door? Well, it's time to get over that and go get some help anyway.

Sure, there are a few people who got fat for purely physical/health reasons. They are working with their doctor on a sound nutritional plan to remove the weight, and their eyeballs are not the ones reading this right now. Everyone else who is fat got so for some mental or emotional reason. And they need mental and emotional help.

It's not complicated logic: if we eat to fuel our bodies, we stop eating when our bodies have enough fuel. We don't get fat. If we are fat, it's because we're eating for other reasons entirely.

What kind of reasons?

- To "stuff" our emotions: boredom, loneliness, anxiety, grief, anger.
- We hate ourselves.
- We were abused.
- We fear sexual attention from others and want to hide (more on this in the next section).
- We have an eating disorder, with all its underlying causes.
- Our parents were really weird about food and passed that on to us—the Clean Plate Club, using food as a treat, withholding food as a punishment, their own eating disorders, being on a diet all the time, putting us on a diet too early.
- We were poor and hungry before, and now can't stop eating in fear of doing without.
- We're all messed-up by the images of feminine perfection we're bombarded with in this culture, and have given up entirely since we feel we can never attain that airbrushed illusion.
- We want love, and somewhere along the way food started to feel like a substitute for love to us.

The possible reasons are endless. You need to know your reasons. More than that, you need to do some healing work with your reasons. If you don't, it's like the foundation of your house has tilted and all the furniture is piled up on one side. By losing the weight, you've rearranged the furniture, but you haven't straightened out the floor. So you're stretched across the floor of your house, your head holding the sofa in place, your hands on the end table and the recliner, desperately working to keep everything where it belongs.

You will fail. You will become tired. You will let go and the furniture will slide back against the picture windows, and you will overeat again until you are fatter than the last time.

Therapy lets you straighten out the floor.

You need to stop fighting the same battle over and over again. Change the terrain. Get underneath the symptom, the overeating, to the cause, the original trauma/pattern.

Get some help. You'll be glad you did.

Sexual Violence Issues

Some form of sexual violence, or at the very least sexual pressure or intrusiveness, happens to every woman in our culture. I can't speak to the male experience, but I would feel safe in saying that a great many of them have been affected by unwelcome and invasive sexual attention as well.

What do I mean by sexual violence? For the context of this discussion about weight, I mean any of the following:

- Childhood sexual abuse
- Adult sexual abuse, coerced sex by a partner
- Incest
- Rape
- Catcalls on the street
- Sexual harassment
- Unwelcome sexualized comments about one's appearance
- Groping, grabbing
- That moment on the dance floor when a stranger holds you too close and you don't feel you can get away without causing a scene

- Bullying or abuse for being differently gendered, a tomboy, or not pretty enough
- Negative consequences for not putting out—physical, verbal, or emotional violence, withdrawal of love and affection
- Being photographed, spied upon, or stared at in an unwelcome sexual way
- Men exposing themselves, suggestive crotch-grabbing
- Being followed, loomed over, or cornered, with a sexual intent

These things affect us in different ways. Not everyone is abused as a child or raped, and those horrors are more likely to damage someone deeply than a catcall on the street. But all of us are different, and our sexual pain is real even if it's not as high drama as someone else's. For someone vulnerable to it, a moment of being taunted sexually on the subway could leave her with a powerful lingering fear of men just as strong as that experienced by a rape survivor.

As women, it never ends. There are moments of unwelcome sexual attention that come our way all the time. You are never too old or too young, too fat or thin, too pretty or ugly to avoid it. There is no combination of dirty hair and sweat pants that will prevent all unwelcome sexual attention from coming our way. There are things that can reduce it, but never eliminate it.

For those of us who are affected strongly by this and seek to avoid it, what steps do we take? Dirty hair and sweats, baggy clothes, no makeup, masculine style clothes, always traveling with a friend, getting walked to our car at night, not going out at night, not going out at all, carrying pepper spray, putting extra locks on the door, learning to glare, cultivating a hard exterior, and best of all... getting fat.

Fat works wonders. It eliminates over 90% of the bullshit. When I got thin again, it was shocking to me how many different strategies I had to re-cultivate for shedding unwelcome males without drama. They approach me all the time, and they all have to be managed or deflected in some way. It's a surprising amount of work. The contrast from not having to engage in it hardly at all and then just six months later having to do it all the time was illuminating. It's a lot of work to be conventionally attractive and safe.

I have more fear now. I am more likely to ask for an escort to my car. I am more concerned about men on the street. And it's not because some overt violence has been done to me since I got thin. It's because these little acts of intrusiveness happen to me all the time.

Don't get me wrong, I am a girl who loves male attention! I thrive on it. I dress to attract it. But when a man has been gently avoided and persists, that's not welcome, even for me.

So. We have all experienced sexual trauma of some form or another. For many of us, this is a key component in why we've become fat. It's just safer, easier, not to be so conventionally attractive.

This works against us when we want to lose weight. Losing weight means taking off our armor—highly effective armor that has been protecting us for years. As the weight comes off, people start making comments about our appearance all the time, like it's any of their business. With every pound, the number of men who approach us increases. It's uncomfortable, strange, exciting but frightening. We feel exposed and vulnerable.

Because we are.

It's not just in our heads. We are actually more exposed and more vulnerable when we make ourselves attractive to a higher percentage of the population. This isn't something you get to wish away.

What is the answer?

First of all, therapy. Talking out past sexual trauma with a professional is essential. It's a whole lot easier to heal, and to stop needing to protect an old wound, when that wound has gotten some first aid.

Second, strategies. Figure out what bothers you, and then think of ways to handle it. If it's streets at night, then plan ahead for an escort. Ask someone to walk you to your car. If it's being approached in bars, wear a wedding ring or take along a friend. Brainstorm. Ask your thin friends how they handle similar situations.

Be very conscious that you feel uncomfortable for valid reasons, and you have to actively intervene or those reasons will take you right back to fatness. The reasons are from the past (therapy) and the present (strategies). Heal and prepare.

You deserve health. It's a dangerous world, and it has hurt you in the past, but *do not let that stop you* from becoming whole and free. Please.

Shaking Fat Person Syndrome—Taking Up Space

A lot of heavy people have what I call "Fat Person Syndrome." It's that belief that they're not worthy that makes them slouch through life trying to be invisible and not take up any space. Many fat people even buy tiny cars—have you noticed this?

Let me assure you of two things: 1) slouching and trying to hide does not make you any less fat, and 2) being fat does not make you any less lovable, no matter what our culture tells you.

This is a problem that has to be attacked on two fronts. Taking off some of the weight can definitely help you feel better about yourself. When we're thinner, we naturally want to show off for the camera, go out more, ride on amusement park rides, and insist on a decent table at a restaurant.

But what if those natural impulses are at war with an inner belief that you're not worthy? If you don't address the self-loathing inside that made you believe you needed to hide from the eyes of the world, there's a conflict. That conflict will inevitably lead to regaining the weight.

Answer any/all of these questions. Write down your thoughts. Discuss them with your therapist or a dear friend:

- Why do you feel unworthy?
- Who told you you were unworthy of love?
- What painful events in your past led you to start hiding?
- How did hiding serve you well in the past?
- Did it create safety for you, help you avoid unpleasant situations?
- How did hiding disserve you in the past?
- Did it deprive you of chances to enjoy life with others, to get up and celebrate the dance of life?

What would happen if you stopped shrinking away from attention? You might be surprised. When I was in high school, I was 40-45 pounds overweight my senior year. Another girl was a good 100 pounds overweight. I had Fat Person Syndrome, and she did not. Guess who took more grief? I did. Me, with my shame, self-loathing, and attempts to hide, got mooed at in 6th period. She, with her bad skin, extra weight, confident attitude, kindness to others, good cheer, and head held high—no harassment I ever saw from anyone who knew her. Hating myself just encouraged others to do the same.

There's a saying, "No matter where you go, there you are." The same is true of weight loss. You can change the physical conditions of your body, but that won't change the emotional landscape within. For that you need to do the work. For that, you need to learn to love yourself.

And buy a big damn car.

Don't Develop Any New Eating Disorders

You've been overeating for years. Maybe you're a compulsive overeater, maybe you're not. Maybe you view yourself as having an eating disorder, maybe you don't. Maybe you have experienced bulimia or anorexia as well.

Whatever the case, there's been something out of control about your eating or you wouldn't be overweight. Turning this around involves gaining control over your eating.

Eating disorders tend to have a strong element of control in them. For many anorexics and bulimics, for example, food and weight become areas of their life they can control in the face of other unmanageable elements.

Compulsive overeating is characterized by a feeling of being out of control when eating. When you find a diet and stick to it, it's a lovely, miraculous feeling to have the cool wind of control come into your life.

Don't get too enamored of it. Yes, control is important. But so is health and moderation. Stick to your medically sanctioned diet/food plan, rather than continuing to restrict things to eat less and less. Let your body handle digestion and elimination on its own, rather than abusing laxatives. Learn healthy eating habits rather than taking weight loss pills.

Watch for warning signs. If you're taking laxatives every Sunday night because you weigh in on Mondays, that's not okay. If you're hiding your eating behaviors, that secrecy could be a sign that you're on the wrong road. If you're eating less than your diet suggests, get back on your diet. If you're at a healthy BMI but still seeing yourself as fat, you should probably get your doctor's opinion and take their advice about whether it's time to stop losing weight. Over-exercising is another warning sign of an eating disorder.

Being in control of what you eat can be a rush. Losing weight can be addictive—there's a great high from seeing that lower number on the scale every week. But you have to keep it in perspective.

Continue to talk to friends, family, your partner, your doctor, or a therapist about what you're eating and how you feel about it. Get the feedback from others about your weight and progress. You can't let them make your decisions for you, but you can let them be a mirror if you suspect you might be getting too extreme in your behaviors.

Don't trade in an old eating disorder for a new one. Find a healthy middle path.

Choose Your Transfer Addictions Wisely

On a lighter note, yes, many of us have been addicted to food in one way or another. Food has taken up a lot of our time: thinking about it, planning what to eat next, shopping, cooking, restaurants, savoring the meal.

Suddenly it's taking up less of our time. It's not being the focus of our attention. Worse, it's not performing its old function anymore, as a cure for boredom, loneliness, anger, grief, etc. Now what do we do with ourselves?

We need to find transfer addictions. Have you ever noticed how many people at AA meetings smoke? They've transferred one addiction to another. Yes, of course, we should endeavor to cure ourselves of having addictive personalities at all. But not only does that sound like hard and boring work, it may also be completely futile. So whether you call them "hobbies" or "transfer addictions," you need to stay on top of the selection process.

If you let them choose themselves, who knows what you'll end up with? A gambling problem and a thing for Vaseline? It's no good. Pick your own.

I went with shopping first. I was somewhat careful to pick stores I could afford. I didn't bankrupt myself. I did spend a lot of money, so perhaps it wasn't a perfect idea. But it worked with my diet. I walked for hours, looking at clothing I could now fit into. I got to reward myself for becoming a smaller size. I repackaged myself, showing off my success, which got me lots of compliments that then fed my resolve to keep going to goal. It worked out.

For a while I tried dating. It was great distraction, keeping several men going in rotation. Unfortunately I have a monogamy problem, and before you could snap your heels three times I'd decided that one of them was the keeper and jettisoned the rest. For a while I had a whole lot of fun with the keeper. The problem with dating as the transfer addiction is that it requires the cooperation of other people, and dating lives have breakups and dry spells. But I don't regret giving it a try.

I also garden, go out dancing (psytrance is my latest obsession—it makes me jump up and down a *lot*), camp, clean my house, cook healthy food, write, play around on the internet, and go to school.

You need to decide what you're going to do with your extra time and energy. As you lose weight you'll need less sleep and you'll want to be up and around more. Take swing dancing classes, join a hiking club, research your genealogy, start a business, or go to Brazil. Whatever you choose, just don't have it revolve around food, and don't pick something unhealthy.

If you want to start smoking or anything else bad for you, know why you're doing it. You've cut off one addictive avenue. Don't let your subconscious drive you down a road that's going to involve another unwholesome withdrawal period later. Steer yourself to something that is unlikely to do you any harm.

And then have fun!

Do Whatever it Takes to Get Whole

Yes, there is something broken inside us. We don't get to where our fat is making us crippled and miserable without having something broken inside. There are a whole range of things it could be—external, internal, spiritual, emotional, mental, past or present.

It doesn't matter what it is. No matter what it is, you can find a way to heal.

I just read an article about a journalist who used very violent sex to heal her PTSD. Does that make *sense*? Maybe not. Would her therapist have recommended it? Almost certainly no. Did it work for *her*? Yes.

I'm not saying you need to get that extreme. What I am advocating is an extreme commitment to fixing yourself.

Is what's broken outside you, in the current shape of your life? Then get a better job or break up with your crappy boyfriend. Move to a house without abusive neighbors. Whatever it is, take one small step every day to turn it around and get it out of your way.

Is what's broken inside you? Track it down and do *whatever it takes*. Seriously. Whatever it takes. Think about what those words mean.

What are your alternatives? Are you happy? Are you as happy as you want to be? Do you feel free of mental/emotional shackles and able to step freely towards the life you want?

No?

Then it's time to get creative. First do some sleuthing. Take an honest self-assessment look at your life, body, mind, emotions, and soul. Where are you disconnected? What are the tender places you shy away from? Where does your loneliness, grief, or anger live?

When you have a list of the things that feel damaged inside and outside you, take a deep breath. Look at the list, and let one item jump out at you. It may be an easy one, a baby step, like getting better shoes so you can go walking more. It's okay to start building momentum with little foundational successes. It may be a harder one, like getting right with God again, that feels huge and makes you cry to contemplate but you know is the cornerstone you must have before you can move forward.

Take that one broken piece of you, and love it. It is you. It is perhaps the best of you. It has made you essentially yourself, human and flawed. It has crippled your progress so you can grow stronger in adversity. Bless it.

Ask it what it needs in order to be released. Brainstorm. Ask friends for ideas. Maybe going back to the church of your youth is too painful, but you can go to a temple first, to start reaching out a hand to the divine. Maybe you can't afford therapy for your self-esteem issues, but you can work through a self-help book. You can't go back and give yourself a happy childhood, but maybe you can buy coloring books and watch cartoons and love yourself.

Anything can work. Healing is a hologram. You can come at it from any direction. The direction doesn't have to make sense—just give it a try and see what happens. The trick is to move energy in the direction of the problem. Give it your attention and love, and magic will happen.

If the first thing you try doesn't work, keep going. Take another step. Try another tactic. Do not give up. You can change your life. *You can radically change your life.*

I believe in you.

Believe in yourself, and do whatever it takes.

VII. SUPPORT FOR THE JOURNEY

A smart man learns from his own mistakes. A wise man learns from the mistakes of others.

Role Models

There really are people who have done it. They have lost 50 or 150 pounds and have kept it off. They have radically changed their lives. Best of all, they know how they did it.

They can tell you:

- The diet they used and why it worked for them.
- The diets they tried that didn't work for them.
- What changed in them between being unsuccessful and successful.
- What pitfalls to watch out for.
- When you're talking like an addict and need to have some sense beat into your head.
- What it's like being thin after being fat for a long time. They can describe the joy, the freedom, the energy, the *life* they have access to. They can inspire you like nothing else, until you have your own successes to keep you motivated.
- Tips and tricks for filling snacks, strategies to make it through hungry days, warnings about whose diet salad dressing tastes like Vaseline, and how to really liven up a diet shake with some sugar-free salted caramel syrup.
- How a thin person orders in a restaurant and avoids the buffet at cocktail parties.
- That you're not alone. They can reassure you that the isolation, fear, anxiety, panic, or sadness you're feeling is totally normal.
- To believe in yourself.
- That change is possible.

You need these messages and information. Trying to change from a fat person to a thin person is an incredibly difficult undertaking. It involves rearranging all of reality in your head, as well as making big changes in the physical world. It's hard to keep the faith.

Role models who have walked this road before you can make the difference. They're not hard to find. They're on the discussion boards of any of the big diet programs or sites. They're there giving back to others who are where they used to be. It's the same urge to extend a helping hand that makes people be sponsors in recovery programs.

Take the helping hand. Thank them for their advice, even if you aren't really ready to hear it. If you don't like the advice, remember it's not an attack. It's intended as help. If it's not the help you want right then, that doesn't make them wrong.

Do you remember any previous times when you were stuck in something unhealthy for you? Remember how invested you were in whatever self-destruction or addiction you were acting out? That's often true for fat people as well. There is a lot of abuse hurled at the "vets" by people who are just starting out with their recovery—or hoping for a magic pill and not actually in recovery at all yet. Don't abuse them, because you *will* want them later. Remember the mood swings and psychotic bitchery discussion from Chapter Six, and try to keep yourself in check.

Thank them as often as possible for showing the way. Their presence in your life is a gift.

Scared Straight

There are some truly gorgeous train wrecks in the world. This is great news. The even better news is that they are utterly willing to spill their crazy all over the internet.

You need the support of watching other people do it wrong. Their failure is your teacher, your mirror, your object lesson in what not to do. It's powerful and wonderful stuff.

People who are busy staying fat will demonstrate all the things one does to stay fat. Seeing these things from outside can help us see ourselves in a visceral, sometimes shocking way. People busy staying fat:

- Open their mouths and give the most hilariously untrue justifications for their eating. "I worked out today," as they eat a bucket of fried chicken. "I have low blood sugar," as they eat a dozen donuts.
- Pretend no one knows they're fat.
- Squish into clothes that are way too small for them. They say things like "these sizes run small, I'm really a 12."

- Avoid situations that will force them to admit fatness: amusement parks, planes, having their picture taken...
- Untag themselves on Facebook.
- Get angry—very angry—at people who try to suggest a better road with less fatness on it. They pick fights on the internet. Lots of them. Their powers of misdirection are epic. It's not about you saying that perhaps peanut butter doesn't need to be on their diet and them disagreeing. No, it's really about what a big meanie you are, and did someone just say "Nazi"? Yes, yes they did. And no, that did not end it.
- Believe in the power of tomorrow to be the day they'll start their diet.
- Pretend they're on their diet, as they're reaching for the bread basket or eating a "salad" with more crap on it than a loaded baked potato.
- Hang out with other practicing overeaters.
- Always have an excuse for not moving—their bad feet, the long day at work, they're just tired, their high blood pressure.
- Blame others for their refusal to change or failure to stick to their diet. Someone made them so angry they had to bake, or they were out with the girls and just had to have a margarita. Helplessness is so attractive.
- Pretend they like their body the way it is. Yes, absolutely you can be fat and beautiful and happy with your body, don't misunderstand me. But people who are busy staying fat when they shouldn't be will claim to be fat-positive, all the while trying to blouse out their shirt to hide their muffin-top and avoiding cameras and fun. There's a difference between genuinely loving your larger body (yay!) and cloaking your self-loathing under fat-positive rhetoric (boo).
- Tell you what an addict they're not. "I'm not a food addict or over-eater, I just..."
- Have a "thyroid condition." No, they're not on medication. No, their doctor hasn't been involved in this internet self-diagnosis.

- Take a "break" from their diet for a holiday, special event, trip, or because KFC released a new sandwich. They plan to get right back on track tomorrow.
- Are "only human." (Insert ranting here.)

This is great stuff, folks. Hanging out on the weight loss discussion boards watching all this unfold was the most amazing gift. It let me see these behaviors and thought patterns in myself. Scared straight? Hell yeah.

Where do you go to find perpetual fatties to be your teachers? Your coworkers, friends, relatives, or people you find on internet weight loss sites. Seek them out. How do you identify them? 1) Fatness, and 2) when the thin people say "don't do that" they say the opposite. If someone is saying something that sounds too good to be true, I promise you it is—it's enabling crap from one junkie to another. Hooray for spotting it, and add them to your list of scared-straight teachers.

Don't ask their advice, or if you do, for sure don't take it. Watch, listen, and learn about yourself.

Support and Accountability

You are going to need support from people who are walking the same road. You need the comfort and companionship, so you have someone who will really get it when you tell them you avoided the appetizers at a party. Sure, your best friend will make supportive noises. But unless she's on the same path she is not going to be able to understand the depth of your struggle, the strength it took to pass a hurdle, the crippling shame when you stumble, or the way realizing you can't shop at Lane Bryant anymore made you burst into tears in the mall.

You definitely want fellow losers to give you support.

You also want them to help keep you accountable. If you're checking in with others, it's harder to lie to yourself. It's also great feedback—you do well, you lose weight, and people celebrate your success. This sets up a positive feedback loop that encourages you to succeed some more.

Hanging out with a community of people who are losing weight together helps you shift your worldview. It serves the same function as AA meetings. People who get your jokes, share your pain, and are working just as hard as you are.

Most people are going to fail in their attempts to lose weight. Not only will most people fail to take it off in the first place, but 95% of people will not keep it off for a year. So my most important advice for you in setting up support for your weight-loss journey is to not make that support dependent on any one person.

If you have one weight-loss buddy, what happens to you when they stop showing up for your morning walks or land face-down in a plate of Twinkies? You think you might find that demoralizing? Yeah, just a little.

Spread it around, or pay for it. Spreading it around means finding a large discussion community online or a weekly meeting. There need to be enough people in your support network that the loss of one or eighteen still leaves you with a community of losers all heading your way. Tons of places exist to find this for free online or through Overeaters Anonymous meetings. You can pay for it by joining a weight loss center with weekly weigh-ins, or hiring a nutritionist or personal trainer.

However you go about it, just make it happen. You will be more likely to stay on track with support. You will feel less crazy and alone. You will get the regular inspiration of others calling out "GOAL!!!!" You will have more *fun*.

Let Your Support Support You

I don't know about you, but I suck at asking for help. I hate it. Deeply, fundamentally, hate it. I'd rather get a root canal than ask someone for help when I really need it. When someone asks me "what can I do to help?" my knee-jerk answer is "nothing, I'm fine." This is always my first hurdle to clear in setting up a support network. I have to force myself to admit that I'm not an invulnerable island. Yuck.

Let's assume you've cleared this hurdle and have some support in your life. You've set things up so you have a place to share your struggles and successes. You have people to give you a pep talk or attaboy when you need one. Good for you.

Now let them do their job. When you fall off your food plan, don't run away from the people who will help hold you accountable.

In order for it to be support, you have to actually allow them to support you.

Admit you're messing up or about to mess up. Talk about what's happening with you honestly. Getting out of denial is always the first step in making a positive change.

Then what? Take it like a grown-up. Are you going to hear just what you want to hear? No. Are you going to get only the flavor of support you prefer? No. Does that mean you should go on an internet rampage telling 75% of the people who are bothering to try and help you that they're doing it wrong?

No.

No really, stop that.

A lot of people prefer soft words delivered in a gentle tone. They want to hear things like "it's just one day, tomorrow is a new day, the most important thing is to forgive yourself and move on." For all I know that crap may actually even help them. I can't be sure, as I am not one of those fluffy-bunny people, either on the giving or receiving end of support.

Some people prefer to get smacked in the face when they're screwing up. I need to hear things like "no, Freya, you're not actually smarter than the docs at Johns Hopkins." I need to be made fun of. I need people who will get in my face. Otherwise, I will ignore the crap out of you and your fluffy kind words. Kind words are never more powerful than my denial. But someone else, when smacked in the face, will shut down entirely, where soft words will sneak under their defenses.

Bear that in mind. People have different styles of giving support because different people need different kinds of support. It doesn't mean that the direct approach is a personal attack, or that the soft approach is just enabling.

What does this mean for you when you need support? Sift through it. Find what resonates in the "get me off my ass" sense, and ignore everything that strikes more of an "it's all good" or "oh, you make me so angry it's your fault I'm eating the sofa with Nutella on it right now" sense. Remember that everyone is trying to help you. Thank them.

Cultivate the ones who give you support that motivates you. Suck up to them. Befriend them. Correspond. Keep track of their kids and vacations. Keep them close to you, as they are invaluable assets.

People who can help you stay out of denial are worth their weight in gold.

And then keep showing up. Post truthfully. Share at meetings. Call your coach. Bust yourself. Don't just drop off the radar because you've been off your diet a couple days. Give yourself a chance to do better, by giving your support network a chance to help you course-correct.

You went to all the trouble of assembling the support, right? So take advantage of your labors. Reach out.

We're here. And we want to help.

VIII. BEFRIENDING YOUR NEW BODY

Yes, I've ruined my body. So what? At least I look awesome in clothes.

Your Jiggly Floppy Body is Funny—Laughter Helps

So you've wrecked your body. You're never going to look like Angelina Jolie naked. So what?

Seriously, so what? You were never going to be as smart as Stephen Hawking, as athletic as Lance Armstrong, as famous as Neil Armstrong, or as kind as Mother Teresa, either. You managed to let all that go somehow.

It's time to let go of the dream of the perfect body. Our media is very intensely bent on the idea that you should hate your imperfect body and keep spending lots of money to try to be less flawed. Allowing our media to control your self-image is not going to serve you well, though.

You will not be able to regain perfection. Stretch marks are forever. Surgery has side-effects, risks of scarring, and creates its own weird things (who doesn't love a vagina that stretches up to your belly button after a tummy tuck, really? I want one of those!) You are older than those models and your youth is never coming back either.

That's the bad news. The good news is that no one cares but you. Or if they do, they're judgmental shallow people who should also go on the list of things that aren't serving you.

Wouldn't it be better to just embrace your body as it is, good and bad? It's all you. Your body shows the history of your life, the adventures it has had. It shows the battles you've lost with food, and now the battles you've won. It's yours.

Own it.

I really enjoy making fun of myself. I called myself "skinny-fat" because although I looked little in clothes, I had all this saggy skin and lack of muscle tone. My friends and I referred to my belly as "my situation." I'd be in the dressing room with a friend and we'd agree "that doesn't work with the *situation*."

My favorite was the day I realized that my situation had some unique properties in water. When soaking in the tub, fatty bits float. Our boobs drift up towards the top of the water. But my belly situation was comprised of loose skin with less fat in it. It didn't actually float. What it did was turn into silly putty. I could squish it into configurations and it would stay there.

The next time my best friend and I were in a hot tub, she made a smiley face in my belly skin. We laughed until we were purple. We horrified the other people in the tub with us. But it was healing for me. It is good to joke about the jiggly bits.

It's like farting during sex. What are you going to do, burst into tears and run from the room, never to have sex again? No. You laugh about it and move on. What are you going to do about being squishy and flawed? Curl up in a ball and die? Save every penny you ever earn for surgeries and potions? Nah. Embrace it and live your life.

Live your life well, and the jiggly bits will be just another thread in the rich tapestry you weave for yourself.

Sagging and Stretch Marks

People who are contemplating or starting a weight loss program ask this question all the time. "How bad will the sagging be?"

Okay, yeah, it's going to be bad. Your belly, thighs, boobs, and upper arms are never going to look like they did before you gained and lost a bunch of weight (repetitively for many of us). But I promise you two things: 1) it will never look as bad to other people as it does to you, and 2) it's still better than staying fat.

So what if you have a bit of a "situation" when naked? How much of the time do you actually spend naked? The rest of the time, you just dress to enhance your attributes and minimize your flaws, *the same as every other person on the planet.* For a saggy belly and thighs? You'd be amazed at how much can be smoothed into place by a simple pair of tights—or Spanx if you're feeling industrial about it. Upper arms? Just wear sleeves. Boobs? Get a bra that fits correctly, and no one need ever know.

Or don't. You'll need to decide what you really want to hide away, and what you just let hang out there. Someone who is comfortable with the body they have is sexier than someone who hates theirs, every time, no matter how normatively pretty they are. If you love and accept yourself, and walk with a sexy strut, your milkshake will bring the boys to the yard. Even if it jiggles.

At this very moment, I'm six pounds up from goal. This is outside my official maintenance window, so clearly I've strayed from the path and am working on correcting that. But aside from that, it's interesting how I feel about my "situation." My worst skin area is my belly. At six pounds up, the skin is more filled out, rounded and prettier. I feel sexier naked. However, I am too muffin-toppy to wear my goal jeans, which is uncool.

I guess what I'm trying to say is that I feel you on the fear of the saggy skin and the dislike of its appearance on the body. But I still want to wear my goal jeans. I am going to take these six pounds back off, and deal with the wrinkly sag. Because most of the time, I'm in clothes, and I like the lean silhouette.

So what do you do about it? Take care of your skin. I have much less of a situation than one would expect after losing 100 pounds so quickly. My skin routine involved regular soaking in the tub and then scrubbing off the dead skin, and lots and lots of moisturizing. Every morning I put on heavy massage oil as I got out of the shower. Almost every night before bed I would cover myself in cocoa butter, shea butter, vitamin E lotion, Vaseline Intensive Care, or whatever blueberry-scented body butter had been on sale at the discount grocery. Yes, my sheets were greasy for most of a year. It seemed worth it.

Other skin routines involve dry brushing, binding with ace bandages, expensive creams of disputed value, sauna/steam sauna, body wraps, etc. For the creams that claim to get rid of stretch marks, be skeptical. The stretch marks are composed of rippled, discolored scar tissue, and unless you have a large pile of money to throw at them, you are going to keep your old stretch marks. Embrace them as "battle scars" and wear them with pride.

Exercise, especially weight training, is a powerful way to help with skin sag. The skin isn't as floppy when it has more muscle to adhere to (or something like that). Many people achieve amazing results with their skin by having a good toning program at the gym. Me? Not so much. I'm letting time and the exercise I get having fun do their best to correct things.

There are many ways to take care of skin. Pick some that work for you and stick with them.

Then try to let go of your emotional attachment to achieving perfection. Aim for better, not perfect. Give it time. Your skin will still be shrinking and adjusting to your new size for one to two years after you hit goal. Give it cocoa butter and let it do its thing.

You do not have to be perfect to be beautiful. You do not have to be perfect to be sexy. All you have to do is be healthy and accept yourself as you are.

I *know* you can do that.

Weird Physical Changes

Losing a ton of weight is a damn strange process. It's like the changes of adolescence, when your body becomes this alien thing you don't recognize. It's like aging in reverse, very quickly. You will have moments of vertigo, a strange panic, when some of these changes come into your consciousness.

Know you're not alone. It is weird. It is alienating. Staying fat is not the answer.

What are some of these weird physical changes?

- The day your hands don't look like your hands. You look at the ends of your arms and don't recognize the parts of you that type and open car doors. You keep catching glimpses of them, and it freaks you out, and so you try to pretend that they're not there looking like someone else's hands, and we can all imagine how easy it is to avoid looking at your own hands.

- Popping joints. My shoulders and spine still pop most mornings on waking. My entire skeleton is trying to readjust itself to not having to hold up 100 more pounds. It doesn't hurt, it's not a joint problem, it's just a prolonged readjustment with sound-effects.

- Reverse growing pains. Things ached as they sorted themselves out.

- Shaving cuts. Seriously. Our legs get angles again. We have bony places, hollows behind our knees, tendons that stick out. It sucks learning or relearning how to shave all these contours after having nice smooth puffy legs to shave for so long.

- Strange bumps. When I make a fist, there's a place just above my wrist that pops out. It's like… a *muscle*… or something. One woman was in the shower and discovered these strange bumps in her throat. She had a moment of despair, that after all this work to lose weight and get healthy, now she's got cancer. After freaking out for a bit, she realized these bumps were the collar bones she hadn't seen in thirty years.

- Sitting hurts. Sitting on benches, the ground, floors, even sitting on padded office chairs – it all hurts. I had to buy a pillow to put on top of my previously comfortable office chair. Did you know there are bones in your ass? Me neither!

- Random painful surprises. You know how when you're having a little kid moment you might knock your feet together, swinging your legs like a child? I did that and hurt myself. My ankle bones knocked together. Really? Bones can run into each other like that?

- People picking you up. At least in my circle of friends, anyway. Guys pick me up when they hug me all the time now. I had to remember what to do—and stop freaking out that they were going to destroy their backs.

- Sleep disturbances. You'll need more sleep for a while, and then a lot less sleep. Your sleep patterns will be changed forever.

- Bed discomfort. I used to need a body pillow to support my upper arm and leg while I slept. Partway through losing the weight, I realized the body pillow wasn't helping anymore. Then later, I realized that my mattress wasn't working out. Fat me had worn a trough in the middle of the bed, and skinny me couldn't sleep in it comfortably. I got a new, lovely pillow-topped mattress, and my arm would fall asleep during the night. I had to put four inches of memory foam on top of it for it to be soft enough for my skinny bony body. It's not necessarily permanent that I'll need this level of accommodation, but for sure when you've newly exposed bones, tendons, nerves, etc., there has to be more squish in your life.

- Horniness. Your libido will wake up. 'Nuff said.

- Veins are easy to find. The people who draw blood would very politely lie to me and tell me that my hard-to-find veins weren't related to being fat. But now that I've lost the weight I can see that was a giant lie. They're easy to find again.

- Agitation and restlessness. You'll find yourself trying to create social events that involve walking or dancing instead of sitting still. You'll be one of those people standing up at a party instead of sitting down all night. You'll hear yourself say "let's go *do* something." Your house will get cleaner.

- Being cold all the time. During the weight loss phase especially, it's hard to keep warm. After losing the weight, it's going to take a year or two to reacclimatize to your own climate. I would wear two pairs of tights under my jeans. My electricity usage was forty percent higher than the year before because I ran the heater so much.

- Crashing out. I had to relearn what was too little fuel for activity. I'd go dancing, come home, and try to go to sleep. Instead, I'd be too cold to do anything but lie there in a stupor, wearing pajamas, a cashmere sweater, a fuzzy bathrobe, extra covers on the bed, and the heater cranked up all the way. Hypoglycemic crashing out with a total failure to thermoregulate. I had to learn that the body needs some carbs within thirty minutes of intense physical activity or I will fall into a metabolic pit and be unable to get out.

- Painful massage. Seriously. When you're smaller, all your muscles are right there by the surface. Massage therapists get in there like all the evil of the world is under your shoulder blades. It takes some getting used to, after having everything all nicely cushioned away from their worst.

These are just the things that I've experienced personally. I'm sure there are more I'm not thinking of right now. You'll have your own list.

It's a damn strange process. Embrace it as best you can. Feeling like your body is an alien thing that moved in overnight is normal. Don't let it scare you away from achieving your goals.

Fat Goggles

Fat goggles: you're gonna have them. When you radically change your body, it takes your brain a while to catch up. Like a year or so. Fat goggles are when you continue to see yourself as fat while you're wearing size eight jeans.

It's surreal. At Nordstrom's two months after goal I asked the sales girl if the dressing room mirrors were "skinny mirrors" and tilted a little. She looked at me like I was insane. I was having a moment where I was actually seeing myself as thin, instead of the fat person I usually see in the mirror, and it weirded me out. I needed a reality check. Despite knowing that "size six" is small and I fit in size six, there's a part of my brain that just figures it's size inflation and really the slender people I see are all wearing size zero or something. Doesn't matter that the scale says "healthy BMI": my brain says "fat fat fat."

It also affects functional things, like not knowing what size space you fit through. Moving through a parking lot or a crowd I am still surprised by the tiny spaces I can slide through. It's like relearning how to walk. I'm delighted when I get to follow a thin person through tight spaces, because then I just follow instead of having to do all this thinking about how big I am right now. My brain lies to me about that one, and I'll walk around spaces I totally fit through.

I'm still sure I'm going to crush my guy when I sit on his lap. When someone picks me up into a hug I'm waiting for their vertebrae to snap like twigs.

One night I saw a cute guy walking arm in arm with a chunky girl. I thought, "Oh good! He dates fat chicks—there's hope for me!" Then I realized I was now thin and his openness to larger women didn't do me a damn bit of good. Darn it.

Fat goggles.

Just know that you have them. Know that you're not going to be a good reality check for yourself about your size for a while. Go by your doctor's recommendation for a healthy weight for you, or what your healthy-weight friends say, or pick a pair of goal jeans and know that if they fit then you're doing it right.

Avoid the temptation to nurture this mild, unavoidable case of body dysmorphia into a full-blown eating disorder. Recognize that you're still going to see yourself as fat most of the time, even when thin, for about a year. Accept the moments when the fog lifts and you can see your lovely self as you are as a gift, but don't count on them.

They worked in reverse for you for a long time, too. Remember when you would think your weight was okay, but then you'd see a photo and be shocked, like it was a picture of someone else? That was skinny goggles—your brain being slow to catch up with your weight gain.

It will catch up. In the meantime, pick that one stable fixed measurable thing (a scale number or pair of jeans) and let it be your guide. Be vigilant about your maintenance, sure. But don't let yourself get crazy. It's just your brain doing the silly things brains do.

Getting Naked and Other Epic Feats of Bravery

For some people, this is no sweat. They get naked all the time, fat or thin. People exist who let it all hang out no matter how bad things have gotten.

Not all of us are this kind of person. Some of you never get nekkid no matter what, so you can skip this section. If you avoid locker rooms and hot tub parties, wear pajamas to bed, and keep the lights off for sex, you do not need to confront the fear of people seeing your naked self.

For the rest of us, we're somewhere in the middle. I absolutely spent less time with my clothes off when really fat (whether naked or in a bathing suit). I avoided those hot tub parties. I didn't date for a long time. I was not comfortable with my skin.

That sucked.

But then, my thinner self also avoided being naked. It's not like they issued me Angelina's body when I got skinny. My boobs are no longer perky. I had folds where my thighs met my ass (although given time this has worked itself out). My belly is always the bane of my physical existence—it has never and will never meet even minimal standards of conventional beauty.

If you're anything like me, you've been avoiding situations where people will see your body, whether that means the locker room at the gym or getting into bed with a new lover. If you're anything like me, there is a part of you that wants to be braver and more self-accepting of your body.

So how do we do this? How do we get naked again?

First of all, know that you are your own worst critic. It is never as awful as you perceive. As my best friend told me, "Honey, I see what you're worried about, but it's not as bad as you think." That was the loveliest thing she could have said to me. She validated my reality, by acknowledging that there were problem areas, but she also let me know it was okay to accept it and hold my head up high anyway.

One thing that might help is to consider what kind of a world you want to live in. Do you really want to be in a world where only the perfect people get to have fulfilling sex lives and sit in hot tubs with their friends? How do you feel when you're at the spa or gym and you see a woman unashamed of her mastectomy scar or big belly? I feel proud of her, and so very glad she's not buying into the shame our culture of beauty-worship tries to put on her. I feel proud of myself when I can celebrate the body I have, instead of mourning the perfection I will never attain.

What about sex? I try to avoid wild generalizations, but this one seems appropriate: sex is always better when you love and accept your body. Sex is always better when your partner shows up with their whole self and lets you love, admire, and touch every part of themselves. It is always an interruption in the energy of connection, love, and hotness when someone hates a part of themselves so much they won't let you see it or caress it.

Yes, you can do what you need to do to feel safe. If you're taking baby steps and being in bed is all you can handle, then keep the lights off and declare your breasts a no-fly zone. Do what you need. But be aware that baby steps should continue to be taken towards wholeness. Challenge yourself. Open yourself. Explore.

Try looking at your naked body in the mirror. Instead of listing off all the parts you hate, or refusing to see them, instead love them. Touch each part of your body you usually judge and tell it why you love and appreciate it. This simple exercise could change your life if you really allow yourself to forgive your parts for being what they are.

If you've got a lover who criticizes your body, you need to do something about that. Like get them to knock it off or find a different partner. However, most people, men and women alike, genuinely enjoy their partner's body with all its quirks and flaws. You might find that something you hate about yourself your partner thinks is adorable. You might find that they just think you are sexy as hell, and don't really dissect things the same way you do. Give them a chance to enjoy you.

Get naked. It's hard. It's scary. It will suck at first if you're not used to it. Work up to it if you have to. But find a way to accept and celebrate your body as it is. You will feel invincible when you know you can walk proud without the armor of clothes. Your partner(s) will thank you for showing up with all of you.

Everyone wins.

Okay, Maybe a Little Exercise

They say you get the weight you want from diet, but the body you want from the gym. I did rant in an earlier chapter about how exercise is just stupid when you're really big. Those reasons have to do with blowing out your joints and discouraging the crap out of yourself by changing too many things at once. But as you get smaller, exercise becomes more accessible—even a smart thing to do.

We all know the benefits of exercise. The heart and lungs get stronger, muscles firm, saggy skin tightens up, and definition appears. You start getting bouncy and active, and you hear yourself saying crazy things like "I'm tired of sitting—let's go *do something.*" You run for the sheer joy of moving your body. It lifts your spirits, alleviates the blues, and solves the energy crisis. It's kind of awesome, really.

Is exercise right for you? Yes. Some form of exercise does need to enter your life at some point if you're going to be healthy.

However, it does not need to be the 90-Day Shred-A-Matic or whatever crazed thing people are all fired up about lately. It could be parking a mile from work and walking in. It could be taking your dog to the park. It could be an active sex life (if you do it right!) It could be ballroom dancing, golfing, figure skating, a treadmill in front of the TV, yoga, or working as a line cook.

Different kinds of exercise will shape your body in different ways, sure. Boot camp and weight training would get you ripped. So would joining the Army. Doesn't mean you have to do either, and there is no requirement that you be ripped. You can stay mildly skinny-fat and just enjoy your life instead.

Try different things. You may like things you didn't like when younger. You may have never been thin enough to enjoy rock climbing, and now that your body will balance properly and is small enough to pull up by your fingertips, it could be your new obsession. Play around. Have fun.

That's what this is supposed to be about, right? Having fun?

Surgery, Lasers, and Other Exciting Technology

So you want the magic of modern medicine to repair the damage you've done to your body. Is this a good idea?

The first step to knowing the answer to this question is to wait. And then wait some more. Like a couple years after you reach goal.

Your body keeps changing. I had a lot of "situations" when I hit goal. I had saggy skin several places. By a few months later, some of those places had completely corrected themselves. Others were still changing. They say it takes a year or two for your skin to finish adjusting after you've lost the weight.

You may regain the weight. I hate to put this out there for you, but 95% of people do regain the weight they've lost, and often add some more. You can be in the 5% club. You absolutely can. But you need to prove that you are *before* you get the surgery. Otherwise, you've just made the situation even worse, when you swell up and stretch out your surgically corrected skin. You thought you had stretch marks before? Or even worse—liposuction. Regaining weight after lipo results in really bad fat distribution to odd places like your back, because the normal locations don't have fat cells anymore.

Losing weight is a sprint with everyone you know cheering you on. Maintaining weight loss is a grueling marathon with no cheering crowds. It's freakishly hard. At this writing I am up 6 pounds from goal. I believe I have the determination to take them back off. I am not going out and buying jeans a size larger. But believing in myself and refusing to buy larger clothes are not the same thing as actually proving that I will do it. I have to set a track record: month by month, year by year, that I will live a life of moderation with food and maintain what I've achieved.

One thing at a time, then. First, wait. Second, wait. Third, really *really* prove you can keep the weight off.

Next, research. Here are some suggested search terms, for an image search:

- Bad boob job
- Tummy tuck scar
- Plastic surgery disasters
- Liposuction scars

I'm sure you can think up your own. Just make sure you really understand the risks. The plastic surgeon will show you photos of the best possible outcomes. You need to do the research yourself to understand the worst possible outcomes, so you can make an informed decision. Is it really worth the risks of scars, botched surgery, infection, and even death?

Maybe it is. You might decide that your reward for your hard work is to get that boob job or tummy tuck. You might want the laser thing that helps sculpt off persistent fat deposits. They're inventing amazing new tricks all the time.

Just do it from a place of love. Love your body as it is, please. It's taken you so far. It's hung in here with you through self-abuse and self-deprivation. Plastic surgery can't make you feel good about yourself if you don't already. It can be a thing you choose to improve yourself, but it will not fix a feeling of not being good enough. You'll need to do that on your own.

I think you're beautiful just as you are. I like our imperfections, the road maps of our lives, written on our bodies. Give yours a chance to be your friend.

IX. DRESSING YOUR NEW BODY

I can either eat what I want, or wear what I want, but I can't do both.

Vanity—Hooray!

Most of us have carried a whole lot of shame while fat. We've avoided cameras, dreaded being asked to be a bridesmaid, loathed dressing rooms, and declined invitations to go to the beach.

We've had to deal with plus-sized departments and stores, which are where they keep the garishly-colored giant sacks of ugly. When you're big, the shopping rule is "if it fits and doesn't make me actively throw up on myself here in the store, buy it." So we dress like crap, because the selection is limited and the whole adventure of trying to find things that are reasonably flattering is totally demoralizing. I used to just shop once or twice a year—go buy a bunch of shirts, a few pairs of pants, and avoid the mall entirely for another six months or more.

Those days are over, darlings. It is time to open your mind and your heart to a whole new adventure: vanity.

Bring it on. You are working so damn hard for this smaller body you're now sporting. You going to keep hiding your light under a bushel? Not under a bushel of fat, and not under a fuchsia floral print sack from Lane Bryant, either.

Getting to care about how you look is part of your reward for losing the weight. You can now doll yourself up and actually be happy with the results. Really happy, not "well, it's as good as it's going to get" happy. You can put on the femme, go out, turn heads left and right, and gleefully seek out the photos on Facebook so you can tag yourself.

Don't get me wrong—I'm not saying you have to, or you have to do this all the time. You can wear your sweats if you want to. But do you really want to? Or is it just long habit speaking? What if you dress as though you have nothing to hide and everything to show off?

What if you dress as though you're proud of yourself?

Is that so wrong?

No.

You should be proud of yourself. You've accomplished something phenomenal. Go ahead—get vain. Refuse to wear things that aren't flattering. Get the perfect belt to go with the new dress. Buy jeans with sparkles on them.

Have fun. You earned it.

Hiding is Okay in Moderation

The rest of this chapter is going to be about showing yourself off, so let's pause a moment and talk about the opposite. Yes, it's okay to hide sometimes.

The process of losing weight is crazy. It radically changes your life in many ways. Some of the time we are simply not ready for the feeling of naked exposure that comes from getting smaller.

As we lose weight, people start commenting. Suddenly every conversation we have seems to center around or at least start with how we're shrinking away. That's a lot of focus on the body of someone who has been trying to hide the state of their body for a long time. It's like a cat who's been trying to cover up their poop on the linoleum (by blousing out our shirt to hide our belly), who is suddenly given a litter box, and then everyone is constantly going "yay kitty, good for you, pooping in the box." Well, yes, we are now pooping in the box, but by you saying that over and over and over you're also saying we were really damn fat before.

It's tough dealing with all the attention, because it brings attention to the fatness we weren't proud of, and brings attention to the thinner body we were uncomfortable enough with to hide under a layer of fat. We feel exposed, vulnerable, or objectified.

We also have to deal with emotionally significant numbers. We come up on 200 pounds, and know that when we get to 199 it's a whole different world. We approach the lowest weight we have been as adults, or the weight we were when we got married, or some other significant number. We cross that line and freak out because it's so alien to our self-identity.

It's all exhausting. Really freaking exhausting.

Take a break if you need to. Wear your fat clothes. Wear baggy sweats, no makeup, and your hair in a ponytail. Stay off the scale. Put your fingers in your ears, go "Lalalalalalalalala," and pretend it isn't happening.

Stick to your diet and keep losing weight, but take a break from forcing yourself to confront the physical reality of it. Sometimes you just need to rest in motion, to lay down in the bottom of your canoe as it heads down the rapids unsupervised.

If you want to hide from the attention, do it. Just don't let that urge keep you from your goals.

What Clothes to Buy While Losing

You are going to need a totally different shopping strategy for the losing process than how you shop when at a stable weight. Basically, when you're on the way down, clothes are disposable, temporary friends. They're only going to be with you for a short while, so don't invest and don't get attached. You can view the local Goodwill as a lending library if that helps.

The first thing you need to learn is that you no longer have to buy something just because it fits. This becomes more and more true the smaller you get (up to a point, of course—if you go down to a size zero you're going to have trouble finding things that fit you again.)

Seriously. Sit with this for a moment. You no longer have to buy something just because it fits.

There are going to be boots that zip over your calves. Lots of them. Most of them even. You no longer have to immediately buy that pair that zips, because there will be more. Cuter ones at lower prices. Things will go on sale.

Things will *go on sale*. In your size. There will be cute clothes left *in your size*. On clearance racks. I'm not kidding—it's true!

I have three pairs of thigh-high boots in my closet right now. I bought them because they fit over my thighs. It took until after the third pair before it occurred to me that this was no longer a reason to alert the media. It's not that I regret having them, but I can see how silly it is to own three pairs of thigh-high black boots just because they fit.

I also have about a million pairs of tights. It was winter when I realized that I could now wear S/M tights, as opposed to M/L. S/M is the smallest size of tights. I was nowhere near goal, but I could fit into the same size I'd be wearing at goal. It was the only area of my shopping where I could unfetter myself, and so I bought a lot of tights. A lot. They have an entire drawer in my dresser plus a hanging shoe organizer.

Anyway, in general, when losing, don't spend a lot of money on anything. Don't buy a lot of anything, even shoes. Your feet shrink. It is common for people to lose a half or whole shoe size when they lose a lot of weight.

Also, your sense of style is going to change radically during this process. Your body shape will change, as will your perception of yourself. The things you buy when 40 pounds from goal are not going to be the things you want to wear at goal. You can't just scale things down, either. If you try on something in a size eighteen and think it's cute on you, that does not mean you should also buy it in a size eight so you have one at goal. It might not be cute on you in an eight, or it might be way less cute than your other size eight options when you get there. Avoid the temptation to "buy ahead."

Stay focused on things that fit you now, that are cheap, and are just enough to get you through. Some people go down a size every few weeks, so the clothing situation is really quite temporary.

Before buying anything, make the most of what you have. Wear existing clothes as long as you can. Get a belt with a lot of holes, and use it to stretch the lifespan of your pants. Don't get absurd about it, but do try to make them last. Once you go to a smaller size, those larger clothes are gone forever. Make them work on their way out.

Keep trying on everything in your closet. Try on all the pants, and stack them in descending order of size. The ones that fit you now go on top, the ones that almost fit underneath, the ones that are a reach under that. Every week or two, try on the top pair that almost fits. Do the same thing with shirts, dresses, etc. Believe me, it sucks to realize you skipped over a totally cute item of clothing and missed its window of attractiveness. Better to be organized about it. If you already own clothes, make sure you wear them when they fit!

What do you buy? The smallest thing you can squeeze into without provoking bystanders to call the Camel Toe Police. A little muffin-top is okay, as long as you wear a baggy shirt over it. You have lots of baggy shirts in your closet already, so this is no problem. You don't want to get anything that is nicely tailored to your body now, because it will be baggy in a couple weeks. Go a little tight instead.

Stretchy clothes are your friend for this. Elastic waist bands. Skirts and dresses instead of jeans. Just do us all a favor and don't do the giant shirt with leggings routine. It's not attractive or fashionable. I know it's convenient, but stop it. Really. You can be just as comfy in a pretty skirt out of a stretchy fabric with some nice sandals, as you can be in leggings. You'll feel better about yourself, too, I promise.

You are going to need to replace all your underwear multiple times. This is disorienting as crap. I handled it by going to Costco and buying one six-pack in each size. I stacked them in descending order of size, and when bigger ones got too big I threw them away. No huge investments in lingerie (or anything) until at goal.

I did the same thing with jeans. Different brands of jeans are sized differently, as you know. It's not like I could buy a size ten in one brand when I was shrinking out of twelves in another, at least not without trying them on. I wanted to avoid the eternal shopping struggle of trying to find cheap new/used jeans in whatever size I was at the moment. I still wanted to have pants that fit. I picked a brand—the Gloria Vanderbilt jeans they sell at Costco. I bought three pairs in a size when I was bigger and still avoiding skirts, and then two pairs in a size when smaller as I was showing off my new tights more. Because I only bought the one brand, I knew for sure that a fourteen was larger than a twelve without any dressing room time. Once I got to goal I went back to the normal thing where you try pants on before buying them.

Get bras a little more often than you think you need to. I know that bra you're wearing is still sort of holding your girls on your body. Sort of. But a well-fitting bra can revolutionize your entire silhouette. It can make all your clothes more attractive, make you feel years younger, improve your posture, and get you free drinks. Seriously. Go buy a new bra. You'll thank me.

Overall, just remember that clothes while losing are a stop-gap measure. Your style will change, your body will change, and you will shrink out of everything you are buying while losing. Get just a few things to tide you over to the next size down.

What Clothes to Buy at Goal

I'm not going to try to tell you how to dress, or give a seminar on fashion. There are lots of information sources way more qualified than I am for that. I'm just going to share a couple ideas and strategies that may help you dress your new, slim body.

First of all, take a deep breath. I remember how disorienting Macy's or Nordstrom were when I couldn't shop in the plus-sized section anymore. There were so very many different departments. I didn't have the first idea where to start. Wait, you mean… the whole store? Like *all* those clothes, with a couple small exceptions, will fit me? I'm pretty sure I hyperventilated.

Then I went to the Jones New York section, because they had made attractive plus-sized clothes so I felt comfortable with them. I knew it was a brand I liked. I still have some of their stuff, but I am so glad I branched out.

It took a lot of time in the dressing room to figure out what looked good on me. Going shopping with a friend really helped. Hopefully you have a patient, supportive, fashion-savvy friend you can take to the mall with you. It's great to be someone's Barbie doll. I had a friend who was utterly enchanted by the process of "here, try this on! And what about this one?" She got me to take risks, both in putting things on my body and in buying some of them.

If you don't have a magical friend with available time to shop with you, use the store employees. Go to Nordstrom on a Monday night at 8:00. I guarantee you they'll be bored out of their minds. Find someone who seems helpful and explain your situation, that you've just lost a ton of weight and have no idea what's going to be flattering on you now. They love this sort of project. I have had the best time with excited sales girls helping me with my makeover. Oh, and make sure to get a bra fitting done while you're here, too. Seriously. You need one.

I'm not saying you have to buy your whole wardrobe at a high-end department store. But it's a great place to start, to get a sense of what cut and style will look good on you now.

In general, think fitted. Remember your goal is to show off your accomplishments, not to hide your fatness. Baggy is out, for good. Even on "period days" your bloat is only going to be a couple pounds. What you used to call "PMS bloat" and "period bloat" was in fact the last forty pounds you were pretending weren't there. Once you're at goal, bloat really isn't as much of an issue as you think it is.

Make sure you get at least one pair of jeans that fit like a glove. Jeans don't have elastic waistbands. They keep you honest. If you can still fit in your goal jeans, you're on track with your maintenance. If your goal jeans become a little muffin-toppy and camel-toey, well, time to readjust your food plan.

Remember you have all the time in the world. You're going to stay at this weight, right? So you don't need to buy a whole wardrobe today. You can take your time, picking up a piece here and there. You can wait for the right thing, instead of something that's close enough. Go ahead, get picky. Insist that your clothes all be things you love, that make you feel pretty, that are comfortable and yet show off your assets.

Have fun. Get some clothes with rhinestones, beads, or sequins.
Show off your cleavage or your legs. You look years younger with
the extra weight gone—take advantage of that and dress a little bit
young.

Celebrate. Show off. Clothing is one of the best rewards for
losing all that weight.

Inexpensive Clothes

You need to buy a whole entire new wardrobe, and you just spent
a crapton of money on your diet. It's expensive, no doubt about it.
However, buying a new wardrobe for a skinny person is a thousand
times cheaper than buying a new wardrobe for a fat person.

You know what thrift stores are like when fat, right? Fat people
hate to shop and have a hard time finding things that fit them. When
they do, they wear those clothes until they fall apart in rags. At thrift
stores, you do not find new things with the tags on them, or designer
stuff that was worn once, in any size with an "X" in it.

The good news is that you do find these things in single-digit sizes
and low double-digit. You find them all the time. Thin people wear
things once and dump them at the Goodwill. You can find them
there. All it takes is time, and not even as much of that as you would
think.

At size six, when I go to a thrift or consignment store I go
through sizes four to ten and pull out anything that looks like it
would be pretty on me. I take a giant pile of stuff to the dressing
room and try it all on. Most of it will fit, and some of it will look
good. Then I decide which pieces are actually worth seven dollars to
me, and buy them. It's a truly magical experience now to shop at a
thrift store. I thought I hated them, but I don't. What I hated was
the horribly depressing experience of trying to find anything remotely
decent in a plus size.

Yard sales are now a possibility for you too. At a stable size, you
can buy things without trying them on. A couple bucks isn't a huge
risk for a dress that will most likely fit you, since it's in your size.

Clearance racks are totally your friend. There will still be clothes
in your size on the clearance racks, and they will be cute, too. I
shopped exclusively from clearance racks when I got close to goal. I
went to the cheaper stores: TJ Maxx, Marshall's, Ross, and

Nordstrom Rack, and shopped the clearance. I signed up for the mailing lists for my favorite department stores so I could go to their big sales. For a while, I stopped paying more than twelve bucks for a dress or eight bucks for a shirt. I just had too many clothes to acquire at once.

Don't neglect the junior's and boy's sections, either. I got a couple totally adorable jackets in the boy's department at Costco. Nineteen bucks for a fake leather jacket with a heavy hoodie liner. Warm, durable, and cheap as crap. The junior's section is totally amazing. Their clothes are fun, fresh, and adorable. They're fitted differently, too, and generally fit my body better than the grown-up clothes. You're also way more likely to find good bling in the junior's section, just in case you're interested in such things.

Don't spend more than you have to. An entire new wardrobe is expensive to put together at once, and you need to buy *everything*. Underwear, belts, bras, dresses, maybe even shoes. It's possible that the only thing you can wear from before will be scarves, and you might decide you're no longer a scarf person.

Take your time and explore. You got thin. Clothes are everywhere.

The Time of Letting Yourself Go is Over, Sister. Kiss it Goodbye

When you're fat, there's this big cascade of things that all lead to "why bother?" You know you're not going to wear skirts, so why bother shaving? Your feet need their special arch-supporting ugly-assed shoes, so why bother getting a pedicure when no one will see it? Your eyes are swallowed up in a bunch of fat and you feel hopeless about everything, so why bother putting on makeup?

Well, sure. It's easy to let it all work together: the fatness, the hairy legs, the lazy hairstyle, and the sweatpants.

That time is over now. You've gone and gotten yourself all thin and lovely, and it's important to remember that this change opens all kinds of doors for you. You can bother about many things, large and small, and they will all come together in a presentation that's nothing short of *snazzy* (as my mother would say).

What does this mean specifically? Well, things like heels, posture, makeup, jewelry, fitted clothes, and colors. Let's take each in turn.

Heels: yes, you think of them as little torture chambers for your feet. Yes, they have that potential. But they also look totally awesome and say "sexy" like nothing else can. Plus, they're a fantastic quad and ass workout. You'll get more exercise doing the same amount of walking, just by wearing different shoes. When I was fat, my feet hurt all the time. All the damn time. As I got smaller, I started wearing some shoes without my orthopedic inserts. Then I graduated to cute little kitten heels—training wheels. After that, the smaller I got, the higher my heels, until I'm quite comfortable running around all day in four inch heels, and higher for special occasions. My guiding principle was to keep my foot pain below what it had been at my fattest. As long as my feet continued to hurt less than they had, I could give myself a little pain to train them to handle higher heels.

It worked. My shoes don't hurt me anymore, and I gradually learned to handle higher and higher heels. You should see me do the Charleston in five-inch heeled platform boots—it's kind of impressive.

My point is, consider embracing a little discomfort to get used to more adventurous shoes. They're so pretty, they give you great lines, and they're the funnest things in the whole entire world to shop for.

Posture: almost all fat people slump. It's part self-loathing and shame, with that whole attempt to hide and avoid taking up space thing. It's also partly a physical consequence of a severely overburdened skeleton. It's just not possible to be ramrod straight when your balance is all thrown off by a big belly. It's not possible to hold your shoulders up and back when your arms weigh so much.

Now that you're losing weight, it's time to pay attention to your posture again. Use the time of all these changes to gradually retrain yourself to stand up straight. It'll make your clothes hang better, too.

Makeup: even if you've been wearing makeup your whole adult life, you might need to change up your routine. For example, when our faces are all round, we put blush on the apples of our cheeks. When you unearth cheekbones, you put the blush underneath, to enhance the shadow below. Consider heading down to the mall to get one of the beauty counter women to do your makeup and discuss some new looks. Why not get an update?

If you haven't been wearing makeup, why not? It's fine to be all fresh-faced and hippified if that's your thing. But even fresh-faced hippie girls might want to be able to clean up nice once in a while for a special event. If your reasons for avoiding makeup are to avoid attracting attention, or because it doesn't seem worth the trouble, are you still content with those reasons? Think you might want to show yourself off a little bit?

They make all these amazing lip stains that stay put all day, with zero effort. I have a casual makeup look that's just eye shadow and mascara, no eye liner at all. You can have a quick routine that is easy to maintain during the day, and which will still let you feel your shiny best.

Jewelry: I avoided jewelry when fat. It didn't seem worth the trouble. Rings? Forget it for my puffy fingers. Earrings? Maybe, every once in a while.

As I lost the weight, I started being enchanted by putting together an entire outfit that sparkled and *worked*. Jewelry and other accessories are the finishing notes for wardrobe. You don't have to spend a lot—costume jewelry and consignment stores are your friends.

Fitted Clothes: I discussed this above, but I'll say it again: time to stop wearing burlap sacks. Get clothing that fits you and flatters the figure you have now.

Colors: Remember colors? I know you've been wearing a lot of black and other dark colors, hoping it's "slimming." Well, sure, black may have been more slimming than a floral muumuu. But even more slimming than wearing black is being slim. Now that you are, how about brightening up your wardrobe? Bright colors, prints, even (gasp!) horizontal stripes. The world is your oyster. Have fun with it.

A Hottie Style: how long has it been since you've had a personal style? I know I didn't when I was big. I just wore whatever jeans would fit me, and whatever baggy shirts didn't make me vomit on myself.

Spend some time wandering around the stores, or perusing fashion magazines, and consider what elements you might incorporate into your style. Are you a big clunky accessories kind of girl? Do you design your outfits around spectacular shoes? Do you like to pair up contrasting textures and patterns? Do you prefer bright colors and flowing fabrics, or more austere black and white tailored clothes?

During the winter, I got very into black and gray. I had black and gray sweater dresses, blouses, skirts, and pants. I had a bazillion pairs of black and gray sweater tights, tights, and socks. I'd wear a black and gray sweater dress with black and gray argyle tights and contrasting patterned black and gray argyle socks, all finished with chunky-heeled lace-up vaguely sexy-librarian shoes. It was adorable, if I don't say so myself. I had so much fun just using the same color palette, but mixing and matching the patterns and textures.

By having a dominant theme in my closet, it was very easy to bring in new items and know that I'd have stuff to wear with them. A personal style can be a lot of fun to develop. Give yourself permission to express yourself through your clothing, with whimsy, purpose, class, or whatever qualities you wish to project.

Ditching Your Fatty Clothes

Should you get rid of your fat clothes? Only you can answer that. I recommend some serious soul-searching on this question.

You should not get rid of your fat clothes if you're going to regain the weight. Seriously, this is a real possibility. 95% of people do regain their weight. For individual dieters who are maintaining their goal weights, we hear countless stories about all the times they lost and regained weight over the years.

I was one of those people. My mindset on a diet was never "I'm going to be thin forever." It was always "I'm going to take off a bunch of weight and then go back to normal." Well, "normal" involved slow steady weight gain until the next disastrous breakup, and then it involved intensive dedicated weight gain until the next diet.

I never got rid of my fat clothes. I just packed away the things that still had some life in them, and threw out the stuff that was worn out. When I got fatter again, I'd go to my closet and pull out the things that fit the larger me. It wasn't really conscious, but it was an unconscious acknowledgement that I hadn't changed my underlying eating habits or emotional relationship with food, and I was going to need those larger clothes again in the future. I always did.

If this is you, keep the clothes. If you're not at the "permanent life change" place, don't try to pretend you are. It's unnecessarily expensive. Pack them away, learn everything you can from your current adventures with your weight, and wait for your moment.

Your moment will come. Mine came when I was crying my eyes out after climbing those stairs in Mexico, or maybe when I heard myself say "I don't like to dance." At some point, you'll hit bottom and will truly be ready to change your life forever.

If you're there, ditch your fatty clothes. Get rid of them as soon as you shrink out of them. Close that door forever. If you only keep clothes that fit you at goal, guess what happens when you regain a few pounds? You have nothing to wear. This is highly motivating to take the weight back off, let me tell you. It's a quick wakeup call, an early warning system. Even if you're avoiding the scale or rationalizing what it's saying as water retention, your muffin-toppy pants will force you to pay attention.

There's only so long you can stick to the flowing dresses and stretchy waistbands part of your wardrobe before you admit that your pants don't fit.

And then you get back on your diet, or get strict about your food plan, or whatever course-correction you need to do to get back on track.

Getting rid of the clothes is amazingly liberating. It's an affirmation of your commitment to your health and your figure. It makes the weight loss real, somehow, to see the larger clothes going away. Can you imagine what it would feel like to know there's not a single item of clothing in your house that's plus-sized?

Release them back into the wild. You'll be glad you did. Keep that one pair of fat pants* for your "after" picture of you standing in one leg, and send the rest of it on its way.

*And cashmere. You also keep anything cashmere. Sleep in it, wear it for housework, whatever. You'll never enjoy a wintery night's sleep more than when wearing a baggy cashmere sweater.

X. LIFESTYLE CHANGES

Egg rolls are not more important than dancing.

Having Fun—It's Okay. Really.

For many of us, being fat is a gigantic cluster of things that are not fun. We don't feel good, we don't have a lot of energy, we don't feel sexy, we want to hide our fatness from others, we're not comfortable standing/walking/sitting in small chairs/etc. Our reasons for being fat are also not fun: addiction, abuse, fear, self-loathing, depression, poverty, etc. All of this combines in our brains to convince us we're not really that into fun.

We pretend we prefer the life we're living. We pretend we're just the "stay at home and read a book" type. We pretend that the sofa and TV is how we like to spend our evenings. And the big bowl of ice cream or Doritos does take the edge off the pain, so it's really not that bad.

Or so we try to convince ourselves.

We do a really great job of convincing ourselves, too. We come to believe it. We come to believe that there's something dangerous about fun, that we don't deserve it, and that if we have too much of it we're just inviting trouble.

Guess what? It's time to turn that around. It's time to work that joy muscle, and get it back into fighting trim.

I had a lot of trouble with this. As I lost the weight, I had more energy. Even without changing anything external in my life, I needed less sleep and had more physical reserves. I could go out dancing or socializing and not pay a heavy price in fatigue the next day. But it made me deeply uneasy. I felt like I was waiting for the other shoe to drop, or like I was doing something wrong.

Well, I wasn't. There's nothing wrong with fun. If you've been having too little of it for too long, there's also nothing wrong with a little fun bingeing. Sure, you need to make sure your rent is paid and the kids are fed, but beyond your basic responsibilities it's okay to just celebrate life.

Keep an eye on yourself. If you find yourself saying no to something, ask yourself why. Is it just out of habit? Do you feel you have exceeded some "fun budget" and don't deserve more? Is it something that fat you couldn't have enjoyed but thin you can?

Try saying yes instead. I accepted all party invitations for a while, no matter what they were. I went to a wedding fundraiser party for a couple I'd never even heard of, much less met. I wasn't invited, I just saw the party go by on Facebook and a couple people I knew were going. I had an amazing time, danced my ass off, and am now friends with the couple.

Saying yes can take you some random places. You might decide you don't like some of the things you try. But at least you gave them a shot and learned something about yourself. I promise you—you will love some of the random things you try.

Surprise yourself. Grow your world. Celebrate life and your body.

Have fun.

New Hobbies

I covered a lot of this idea in the section on choosing your transfer addictions wisely. However, I'd like to repeat the idea here: you are going to need to develop some new hobbies.

Knitting while watching TV is a great hobby when you're fat and sedentary. It's not going to be enough when you're thinner and active.

You will have tons more energy. You will probably sleep less. Your body will want to move rather than sit, dance rather than watch, go play rather than zone out. You need to channel this energy into new projects and hobbies.

At this moment, I am repainting the exterior of my house. It never crossed my mind before that I could paint an exterior myself. Turns out it's not technically challenging, just a crapton of hard work. Well, I am totally up for that.

I'm still not in shape to do it for a living, but I can do five-hour work days of manual labor. I enjoy being out in the sun, getting all tanned, feeling the soreness in my forearms and shoulders. I love the feeling of satisfaction from knowing that I'm doing this job well and my house is going to be shiny and gorgeous from my efforts. I know that if I had wood floors in this house I'd be refinishing them next.

Be as creative as you can. Think big. Think active, challenging, and new. Take up rock climbing or hiking. Build a deck. Start a program to tutor immigrants in English. Build a bicycle from parts. Go out dancing.

When you're busy and active, you're also not obsessing about eating. New hobbies are a critical part of your maintenance plan. It all works together.

Accommodations

Your thinness is going to need some accommodations for a while. Things are different. They're pokey, boney, and cold.

What kinds of accommodations do you need? They come in two main categories: protection for boney bits, and warmth.

For the protection of boney bits, I needed a pillow for my office desk chair. Seriously. The padded chair that had been totally comfortable for 5 years was suddenly rock hard and impossible to sit on all day. I had to buy a pillow to make it tolerable.

I no longer sit on the floor without a pillow. I'd rather stand than be on a hard bench or plastic chair. This effect is getting better as I develop butt-calluses or whatever it is that makes your sit bones less hurty, but my butt still gets sore in ways it never did before.

My legs will fall asleep in unpadded chairs or if I sit too long in one place. I was having the problem that both my arms and legs would fall asleep in bed. My old mattress wasn't working for me. I had to buy a whole new bed, plus a four-inch memory foam topper. On that, I'm fine. But it's a lot of squish.

Staying warm was a serious challenge while in the weight loss phase. It's better now, but it's also summer. I may still be a horribly shivery thing next winter—we'll find out.

I had fingerless gloves for work, as well as a space heater by my desk. I kept sweaters everywhere. I wore two pairs of tights over each other inside my jeans. I layered hoodies—sometimes I'd have three hoods inside each other. I live in Seattle—it's not like the arctic—and I remember wearing a hoodie shirt inside a hoodie-lined faux-leather jacket inside my wool overcoat. Who wears a jacket inside an overcoat in Seattle? Crazy people, that's who.

Get an electric blanket or some new down. Make your husband warm up your side of the bed. Wear cashmere to sleep in.

Drink hot beverages. Seriously, it helps. I discovered that just drinking a cup of hot water can make an enormous difference in my degree of frozenness. Yes, the bartender looked at me like I was a nutjob, but at least after I drank it I could take off my gloves inside the bar.

Your life is different in a lot of ways. Remember to change the infrastructure a little to support your new body. Don't be shy to ask your hostess at a dinner party for a lap blanket or a pillow. Get what you need to take care of your pokey bits and stay warm.

Unearthing Your Real Problems

Overeating is a great insulator. Many of us use food to buffer us from our feelings. A nice bowl of pasta can quiet the inner turmoil and get us through another night.

Being fat is a great excuse. We can tell ourselves we're just miserable because we're fat. Once we lose the weight we'll be happy.

I saw this quote recently: "The two hardest things to handle in life are failure and success." Getting close to goal raises all sorts of fears. What do I do now? What comes next? What will I do when I can no longer use my weight as an excuse for not accomplishing things?

Guess what? You lose the weight and you naturally unearth your *real* problems. Turns out you're not unhappy because you're fat— you were unhappy because of X, Y, and Z, and you ate to cope with that misery. When you remove the food, you still have X, Y, and Z, and you've lost your favorite coping mechanism.

First off, this sucks. It totally sucks. I just want to acknowledge that this part of the process is absurdly hard sometimes. It feels brutally unfair that just as you're getting your life together, finally losing the weight and turning things around, you have all these other issues up in your face.

Well, some of them have to be handled for you to be able to have a functioning life. You might need a new job or partner. You might need to create more distance between you and your mother in law. You might need to cancel your credit cards and get out of debt.

Don't be surprised when you find that some areas of your life feel like total crap. This is a natural part of the process.

First, notice the situation and your feelings about it. You might need to talk to someone, like a close friend or a counselor.

Second, wait. The weight loss process has some gigantic mood swings and hormonal shifts. Don't make rash decisions you might regret later.

Third, strategize. What do you really need to correct the situation? Can you negotiate some different communication rules with your partner instead of breaking up with them? Can you transfer to a different team at work instead of quitting? Try to think broadly about all your options. Brainstorm freely.

Fourth, act. Make changes in the real world to change your life. If a situation is dragging you down, fix it. You are no longer going to be the person who puts up with crap in silence, muffling her screams with another plate of Twinkies.

If you are no longer that girl, what does your life look like? Dream up a better life, and make it happen.

Take action *now*.

XI. SOCIAL "ADJUSTMENTS"

Finding out who your friends really are sucks.

When No One Says Anything

Before we dive into a discussion of how to handle it when people won't shut up about your weight loss, let's discuss the (highly frustrating) opposite situation. What do you do when you've lost 20 or 40 pounds and still no one has said a word about it? Are you going to let their silence demoralize you?

No, you are not. You're going to get out your camera, take a picture of yourself, and compare it side-by-side to your before pics. You're going to see for yourself how much you've accomplished, and take great pride in it. You're going to hold your head up high and wait it out until the rest of the world catches up with your awesomeness.

Why haven't they said anything? For a small percentage, they haven't noticed. This can totally happen with people you see regularly. A gradual change like weight loss can sneak up on you like someone going gray. It's a different thing from someone dying their hair purple—we notice sudden, dramatic changes.

It's far more likely that they're not sure if they should say anything. What if they compliment your losses and find out you've lost weight unintentionally through illness? That's even worse than asking a non-pregnant fat woman when she's due. What if they comment and you get offended, and react as though they're calling you fat? This happens fairly regularly, and it's ruined things for those of us who love praise. It's like how a man can get gun-shy about opening doors after being screamed at for it.

Many people wait for your lead on whether it's an open topic of conversation. I would hear a lot of "I love your new haircut" or "you look fantastic" when what they meant was "jeez you lost a lot of weight." They'd have this nervous look on their face. As soon as I said something like "I've been working really hard on taking off the weight" or "thank you, I'm down 40 pounds" they'd chime in with comments like a dam had burst. Feel free to broach the subject first. You'll start to recognize the constipated expression when people are trying to decide if they can address the subject or not.

A few of them are jealous or threatened. You're never going to get a sincere compliment without a backhanded insult inside it from these people. Let it go, and stay on track. This isn't about them.

It's about you and your awesomeness. Go look at those photos again.

When People Won't Shut Up

If you lose a lot of weight, there will be a prolonged period of time where every conversation you have with anyone starts with a discussion of your body.

Let that sink in for a minute. *Every* conversation. Your *body*.

If you've got any urge to hide, inner shyness, shame about your weight, or sense of privacy, this is going to suck pretty quickly. Yes, compliments are great. Yes, some of us really adore them. But even for the attention whores among us, it can get old in time. (Right before it starts to taper off and you miss it like a junkie in withdrawal.)

No way exists to get this to stop happening, so don't even bother trying. You are not going to be able to "put the word out" that you don't want to talk about it. People are going to compliment you, and you need to find a way to put up with it.

My best advice is to accept the praise graciously. Allow them a couple sentences if they're an acquaintance, longer if they're a closer friend. Thank them, mention how hard you've been working or how thrilled you are. Then change the subject.

The easiest subject segue is to counter with a personal compliment of your own. Tell them how wonderful they look, admire their haircut or clothing. If you suspect they're going to be hard to deflect from the subject of your weight, you can move a bit into their personal space with the compliment. Stroke their arm as you admire the fabric of their jacket, for example. Be a little bit too excited about it. The slightly intrusive personal attention will make them uncomfortable, and they'll be more likely to jump on a neutral topic when you present one.

While you're admiring their personal appearance, rack your brain for another conversational sally. Take control of the conversation quickly while they're figuring out what to do with how excited you are with their glasses or purse. Ask them about work, school, the kids, that upcoming trip. Ask follow-up questions. It'll only take a couple minutes to get conversation onto another track and then you can relax.

Sure, some people will come back to it. Some people really want to know what you're doing so they can do it too. Of these people, most of them are just hoping you'll say "I took a magic pill and my ass-fat went to live on Angelina Jolie." If they seem like they'd sincerely do some work, tell them how you did it. Give them the info they need to follow in your footsteps. If they're the lazy dreamer, I loved the answer one woman would give about the Medifast diet: "I'm on a low-calorie, low-carb, low-fat diet." That's just not attractive to most people—one of them they could consider, but all three? Ouch! I would say "I've been living on 900 calories a day for the last six months." That would also shut up most people, unless they wanted to dive in with a lecture about how I was killing myself.

As I said, it's not possible to avoid the topic. Try to handle it with grace and class. Know that most people have good intentions and don't mean to make you uncomfortable. Smile and nod. Say thank you. If it's really weighing you down and making you want to eat so you can avoid all the attention, go talk to a counselor about it. Don't let the congratulations of others make you stay fat. Your health is worth working through this.

Losing Your Fat Friends

Perhaps all of your friends will be staunch supporters and loyal allies as you move through your weight-loss life changes. If your social world is anything like mine, and that of many women I've spoken to about this process, you are going to lose some of your fat friends. Hopefully not many, but some of them. Why does this happen?

First of all, any radical life change can result in some people drifting out of your life. A divorce, a change in income level, a sudden interest in punk rock and tattoos, whatever. Some people were drawn to you when you were one way, and are not going to make the transition to you being a new way. It's not personal, they're just a more limited kind of friend.

For your fat friends specifically, there are a few things that could be going on. I'll work through them from more emotionally neutral to more emotionally charged.

Activity Partners: some friends are people we hang out with for certain activities. As practicing overeaters, we had activity partners for that. We had friends we'd go to the buffet with, or who would eat appetizer sampler platters with us. We'd go to the movies and share a butter-laden bucket of popcorn. We had a variety of activities that involved overeating and sitting down.

If you stop overeating and sitting down, what does that leave for your fat activity partner friends? If you don't want to lose the friendship, you need to actively strategize for things you can still do with your friends. Come up with new ways to spend time together that don't center on food or trigger you to want to eat. Throw a movie night at your house and serve fattening snacks that you aren't tempted by, or just put out a bunch of healthy food. See if your friend wants to go shopping with you instead, or take a road trip.

Don't try to change your friend. Don't try to sell them on your diet or the joys of being thinner. Believe me, they get enough of that in this culture. Avoid putting that pressure on your relationship. If they want any information, they'll ask you.

Be creative and take charge. Don't wait for them. Be active in helping your friendship transition to a new place that works with the new you, and the same them. Remember that just because it was time for you to radically change your life doesn't mean it's time for them.

Denial: your weight loss can force some of your fat friends to confront their denial. This can happen in a lot of ways. The most basic is it makes it much harder to believe that weight loss is hopeless. Whatever place of having given up hope they're occupying is now threatened by you, sitting there breathing, *thinner*. You don't have to say a word or do a darned thing. Your simple existence is smacking their denial in the face.

Then there's how your behavior confronts their denial about their own habits. If you go out to eat with a fat friend, what do you order? Grilled chicken breast and steamed broccoli? And what do they order? You know how bad it looks, seeing all that food arrive. Then they eat it all, covered in sauce, batter-dipped, deep-fried, greasy carby deliciousness. You don't help with the bread basket and yet it's all gone by the end of the meal. Your behavior forces them to see what they're eating in a new light, right next to what you're eating.

Same thing with their habits. If you're always going out dancing and they're in front of the television, your new habits are confronting their denial about their lifestyle. You're making it very clear that there's another way to live. It can make their world seem smaller and more confining.

There's nothing you can do about this, really. Keep living your life. Give them space to work through their feelings on their own. You will lose some of your fat friends because you make them uncomfortable. Others will come around, after they get you re-categorized as a skinny friend.

Feeling Judged: you might actually be judging them, or you might not. Either way, some of your fat friends are going to feel judgment from you. Your decision to lose weight does mean you judge being fat as less awesome than being thin. No point in denying that. At least for yourself, you hold a value that being thin is better than fat.

A lot of people lately call themselves "fat positive" and act like it's a good thing to be large. I believe a couple things about this: first of all, fat discrimination and fatphobia is stupid and people should knock it off. Second, the health statistics are unavoidable—if you're fat, you're killing yourself more quickly than a thin person, all other things being equal. Third, the physical and lifestyle implications of being fat vs. thin are undeniable as well—if you're thin, you have greater mobility, more options, more stamina, and more energy than someone who is carrying an extra hundred pounds everywhere they go. I have not heard a single story from someone who took off a bunch of weight who says "I just wish I had the energy I used to have. I'm so tired of puffing up stairs now that I'm thin."

My point is, even if we dream up a perfect world where there are no negative social consequences for fatness, there are still the physical ones. At the very least, that seems clear. So if you have fat friends who are working very hard to pretend they're just as happy fat as they would be thinner, you are going to bother them. You are going to make them feel judged, because they're so busy working so hard to pretend everything's okay.

You remember what this was like, right? When you turned down invitations to the water park or a night out with the girls and pretended it was because you just weren't that into fun?

There's not all that much you can do about this. Keep letting your friends know you care and appreciate them, and try not to judge. But know that some are going to feel this way no matter what you do.

Jealousy: the green-eyed monster will raise her ugly head. Some of your fat friends are going to be jealous of your success. They're going to drop by with casseroles or candy, too. They'll try to get you back on the fat train if they can, or just hate the sight of you if they can't.

Again, not much you can do. Let them work through it on their own. If they keep bringing food you won't eat, dump it in the trash in front of them. If they make snide and hateful comments, remember it's coming from their issues, not yours. You can avoid them for a while, or ask them to not make those kind of comments to you.

If they persist in being a negative influence in your life, then you can make an active decision to remove them. Just because they're an old friend doesn't mean they're a good friend. Keep assessing the effect people have on you. You have a new life and should be able to celebrate it. If someone does not bring you happiness and you don't bring them happiness, it's probably time to call time of death.

Overall, your weight loss is a massive upheaval in your life and in the lives of all those around you. They've done research about social networks and found that people follow each other. If a friend loses a bunch of weight, it can start a chain reaction of other people losing weight in the social network (as well as the reverse). You are affecting others deeply.

It's going to hurt, a lot, to lose some of your friends. Know that some may come back later when they've worked through things or gotten used to the new you. Most of all, know that it's not about you. Stay on track and let things sort themselves out in time.

Losing Your Skinny Friends

Perhaps all of your friends will be staunch supporters and loyal allies as you move through your weight-loss life changes. If your social world is anything like mine, and that of many women I've spoken to about this process, you are going to lose some of your skinny friends. Hopefully not many, but some of them. Why does this happen?

As I said above, some of these losses will be simply because any life change brings on some attrition in one's social world. What about the rest?

The only reason I'm aware of for why your weight loss makes a skinny friend get weird and stop wanting to hang out with you is jealousy, pure and simple. You stopped being the fat friend that makes them look good by comparison. You are no longer fulfilling your assigned role, and they get nervous.

Suddenly they see you as competition instead. You're in a similar universe of attractiveness, perhaps even getting more attention than they do sometimes.

Have you had a thin friend say "Don't get anorexic" as you're losing weight? This is pure code for "Don't get skinnier than me."

Tell them how beautiful they are. Be patient. Use some self-deprecating humor if that helps. One very pretty friend of mine was acting threatened. I shifted the dynamic by discussing how even though I looked good in jeans my belly fat situation was all jiggly and horrible. I could feel the energy lighten up between us just by giving her something to still feel prettier about. Not that she had any worries, mind you—a gorgeous girl—but my change in relative attractiveness was still making her edgy.

Overall, within your social world, be prepared for shifts, undercurrents, and feelings people have that they won't admit to. Try not to take it personally. Giving people time to adjust to the new you is very important—give them space to catch up to you.

Make sure you have a community of people who are also losing weight who can validate your reality. It's so important to know you're not alone in this socially awkward phase.

Trying to Keep Your Partner

I discussed a partner's reasons for not wanting you to lose weight in the section above on handling a sabotaging partner. They might fear you're going to leave them, want to be able to control you, or simply prefer the body you started with.

Any of these reasons, or others, might cause them to leave you at some point in this process. When you lose a lot of weight, you revolutionize your life. Big changes occur socially, in your moods, in your lifestyle, in the kinds of things you want to do, in the amount of sex you want to have, etc. Not every relationship is going to weather these changes intact.

Do you want it to? Do you want to keep your relationship? This is an important first question to answer. For some people, an unhealthy or unsatisfying relationship is one of the real problems unearthed by removing the overeating and the weight. For these people, being fat is all wrapped up with the unhappiness of a bad relationship. Removing the fat is a way of opening the door to a better life with someone new.

If this is you, be clear about it. Go ahead and make your choices, make the life changes. Don't hang out and torture both of you, trying to force your partner to make the decision for you. If your heart is gone, take your body with it.

What if you want to keep your partner in your life? Make sure that actively working towards that goal is on your short list of priorities.

Remember, you are the one who is making a sudden life change. They are the one who is expected to keep up and embrace the new you. How can you help them through this?

First of all, communicate. Lots. Keep telling them how sexy they are, how much you love them, how thrilled you are to be able to give them this new sexy body to play with. Point out the limber things you can now do and how good sex is feeling for you now. Reassure them, with word and deed, that you are attracted to them and want to be with them. If they're insecure about other men or women, tell them that you're making this change for you, not because you want someone else. Listen to your partner's concerns, and keep talking.

Give them space to be a little weird about you or act out in strange ways. It's a huge adjustment. Expecting them to cheerlead 100% of the time and never have any other emotional reactions is unrealistic. Be patient.

Know that you are changing in more ways than physical appearance. Besides the mood swings, there's also a common pattern of starting to stand up for ourselves more when we stop hiding in all the fat. You're bringing a new dynamic into your relationship. You might be taking less crap, not allowing your partner to take you for granted, or just demanding more psychic space in the relationship. Be patient and supportive as your partner adjusts to this, too. You're renegotiating things mid-journey.

Try to avoid demanding your partner change their lifestyle or weight just because you are. You remember what it's like when other people tell you that you should lose weight, right? How it makes you want to curl up with a pint of ice cream until they shut their flapping traps? Well, don't be that nag. Your partner may well get caught up in your slipstream and start changing their life as well. They might join you on your diet, or get their bike out of the garage to go with you on your new trips. They might not. They might purposefully sit still for a while longer, waiting to see if your love is conditional on them changing the very instant you do.

Don't make your love conditional. Don't expect that the person you got into a relationship with is going to change on a dime just because you are. Make the changes you need to stay healthy, and let them do whatever they do. If you need a biking buddy, find one, but don't pressure your partner.

As Tom Sawyer showed when whitewashing the fence, we get much better results by saying "Party over here!" than we do by trying to browbeat people into doing things. Keep looking like you're having a good time and they may well join you. Worst case scenario: you keep having a good time, and you bring home your bubbly enthusiasm and sweaty limber body to your partner.

Overall, remember that just because your changes are a gift to you, they may not seem like one to your partner, at least not right away. Find ways to share positive time with your partner. Find new activities that work for both of you. Remember that it's not all about you, even though it can seem like it sometimes.

Love them, and do the work.

You Won't Be Invisible Anymore

Despite taking up a lot of physical space, fat people get ignored a lot. It's a shock to the system to find that one is no longer passed over for attention in a variety of social contexts.

I couldn't stop telling the story the day it happened in Home Depot. I was *in* the light bulb aisle, *looking at* light bulbs. A store employee asked me if I was finding everything okay. Walked up to me, and asked me if I needed help. It was amazing. I was no longer invisible.

A lot of privilege comes with being of a conventionally attractive weight. It's a massive shift in social status. People everywhere are going to be more helpful and attentive, and generally more aware of you.

Try to use your powers for good. I had to learn to flirt less. The amount of charm I had to point at someone when I was fat, in order for us to have a fun interaction, was way more than necessary when thin. It feels like suddenly having a superpower. Just as a new superhero or vampire has to learn how to hold his super strength in check, you need to learn just how much eyelash fluttering is necessary or appropriate. Just bear in mind that it's a different setting than you're used to.

Where appropriate, hold a grudge. A guy in my circle of friends acted like I wasn't in the room when I was big. Once I got thin, he started seeing me again. Guess what, dude? It could be *decades* before I acknowledge your existence.

I considered being angry about all the new attention. Why wouldn't people just be decent to everyone they encounter? For me, I feel that rejecting a privilege I have doesn't give it to the people who don't have it. Long, slow work to change social attitudes can eventually result in leveling the playing field. I can make sure that the fat person near me doesn't get skipped over for assistance from a store clerk, but I can't make them be treated the same way.

It is a shocking difference in how strangers treat you when you go from being fat to being of a more average weight. It can be depressing as hell, because it makes it so clear how much attention and respect you weren't getting before. If you can, enjoy the benefits that come to you. If you're inclined, do what you can to buck the trend of ignoring the fat. After all, you know *exactly* what it's like on both sides of that funhouse mirror.

No More Fat Jokes

I hate to break it to you, but your days of cracking fat jokes are over.

Perhaps you're a nice, polite person who hasn't been in the habit of making fat jokes among your friends, or occasionally poking fun at your fatness in front of a stranger or two. If so, please skip to the next section. But if you're anything like most of the people I know, we love to make fun of ourselves and each other with the occasional "that's what she said" or fat crack. We just can't help it.

Well, now that you're all skinny and stuff, this is a *bad habit*. Dangerous. It will make you look like a mean girl.

Case in point: I was on a second date with someone. A larger man. I do like my guys big. We were watching a movie, and on screen the characters were talking about stuffed crust pizza. He said, "I like stuffed crust pizza." I replied, sarcasm dripping, "Shocker!"

Oops. The words were out of my mouth half a second before I remembered that I wasn't fat anymore. It wouldn't come across as jovial joshing "we're all in this fat thing together." Now I'm a snotty skinny chick making fun of the poor fat guy. Darn it.

Luckily he took it in good humor, but I learned my lesson. Remember my audience. I only get to make fat jokes with people who knew me fat, or who know my history and that I have that kind of relationship with. It's really hard to retrain myself, but I definitely don't want to be part of the problem for someone else.

Sigh. It was fun while it lasted. I guess I have to learn how to make jokes about eating a lettuce leaf for lunch or something. Develop some new material.

If you're still big, please tell some fat jokes for me while you still can.

Dating—You Don't Have to Date Them Just Because They Want You

[This section is for the women who've been dating and settling. The next section is for the women who've been waiting for Mr. Right.]

I'm about to horribly over-simplify to make a point so don't come after me with sharp objects, okay? Please?

Attraction is largely instinctive, and a big part of it is our unconscious assessment of the likelihood of raising healthy progeny with the potential mate. This applies whether we plan to have kids or not. The things we find attractive—curves and shiny hair on women, broad shoulders and a confident attitude on men, a full set of teeth and a quick wit on either—are indicators of suitability for child-bearing and rearing.

The same goes for weight. There's a big bell curve laid over the weight distribution, in terms of how many people will be attracted to people at different weights. Put another way, if you're an "average" weight, somewhere in the middle, there are a lot of potential partners. If you're out at the edges, whether very fat or very thin, there are fewer people who will be attracted to you.

It's not personal, it's not judgment, it's not fatphobia or skinnyphobia, it's just an unconscious reaction to your probable fertility.

Of course there are a bazillion other cultural, social, and personal factors that go into attraction. But it all comes down to the same thing—when you lose a bunch of weight, as long as you don't go too far, you will gain many more potential partners.

When we're fat, we're used to scarcity. We are used to being ignored by men. We fear being judged and rejected because of our weight, because we *are* judged and rejected for our weight. As a result, when a man comes along who expresses interest (as long as it's not that creepy "let me feed you buckets of fried chicken and play with your fat rolls" kind of interest), we bend over backwards to be interested in return.

We will compromise the crap out of ourselves. We're so grateful for the attention, thrilled to have a chance with someone, and delighted to not have to be alone, that we will ignore all kinds of things. We'll ignore that we aren't that that attracted, various deal-breakers, bad attitudes, and worse. A certain kind of man knows of and uses this desperation against us.

Some of us give up on dating altogether. Others keep trying, but encounter a lot of disappointment. Some of us end up in relationships that are unsatisfying or abusive. Some of us are in happy marriages, and of course this section on dating is not for you.

If you find yourself single and newly thin, it's a whole new world. Your pool of potential partners is immense. It's like when you are no longer shopping in the plus-size section, and instead have the entire mall. You have a lot more to choose from.

A lot.

The same advice applies that I gave for shopping—you no longer have to buy it just because it fits. You no longer have to date men just because they want you. You don't have to give someone a shot when you can spot a deal-breaker up front or think they smell funny.

You can take your time, consider your options, date around, and have a good time.

Let men take you out and buy you dinner. Make them plan your dates. Have them come pick you up. Sit in the car until they come around to open the door for you. I'm not saying this is the only or best way to treat men, and it's not how I treated the guy I ended up with, but it was so good for me for a while. It was balm for a bruised soul to be treated like I was special by dates. In return, I dressed up with really good shoes, and gave them a shiny pretty girl to show off for the night. Everyone was happy.

Let dating be fun for a while. If one guy doesn't work for you, there will be another. If you get brave and start asking out cute boys instead of waiting for them to ask you, there can be *lots* more. Men usually say yes when you ask them out. It's fun as hell once you get over the panic. Who cares if they reject you? There are so many more where that came from.

Are you hearing me? Many more where that came from. Lots of fish in the sea. Make sure you keep throwing back the little ones until you find one that treats you right and makes you feel like you're home. You deserve it.

Dating—Real Men Fart

[This section is for the women who've been waiting for Mr. Right. The previous section is for women who've been dating and settling.]

Being fat can be like being a princess locked in a tower. There's a great view and a lot of quiet time to read romance novels, but no one can get to you. Many fat women hide away instead of engaging with life. The problem is that thinking about Mr. Right when you're avoiding dating is a lot like planning how you'll spend your lotto winnings when you never buy tickets.

For those of you who've been building up a picture of Mr. Right in your heads, but not getting any practical hands-on experience, it's time to lower your standards and come out of the tower.

Lower your standards a *lot* and get out there! Being in relationships takes practice like anything else. If you stay alone, waiting for some mythical perfect guy, you never get to learn how to be with real guys, with all their farts, stupid jokes, and rough spots.

Leave your standards high in terms of how they treat you—never take abuse from a man. But as for the rest of it? Just date some people. You will learn far more about what you like in a man by being in relationships than you will by thinking about it and making a list. You can't graduate from school without sitting through a lot of classes. You can't find Mr. Right without kissing some Mr. Right Now's.

What we think we want when we don't have relationship practice is a mishmash of things we want and stuff our culture tells us we should want. It's distanced from reality. The only way to bridge the gap is to try things out—and you might surprise yourself. That guy with the "total dealbreaker" thing about him? He might be a wonderful love you will be forever grateful you gave a shot. You might find that you don't mind his smoking, unemployment, age difference, weight problem, or whatever thing you thought at first was a total hard limit.

You can also learn things in the good direction. I would always bitch about emo guys, and say I wanted a nice screwed-up locked-down guy so we wouldn't have to talk about his feelings. Now, I cherish my current partner's emotional directness above any other quality of his, and it wasn't anywhere near my list of things I thought I wanted.

Get yourself an online profile, and then meet men for coffee. Don't correspond with them for weeks or months first, don't talk on the phone, don't quiz them about your deal-breakers. If they're potentially cute and don't seem utterly psycho, ask them for a coffee date and get out of your house. You'll learn more in a half-hour in person about actual chemistry between you than you could in six months of talking.

Ask men out at parties, square dancing, and the Corgi Appreciation Club. Get out into the world, meet men, ask them if they're single, and ask them out for coffee. Keep an open mind. Throw away your long list. If you have more than five essential requirements you're not really looking for a relationship.

Be open to what life brings you. Don't be so focused on God's left hand that you ignore the bounty the right hand is trying to give you. You deserve to live and love. Let it into your life.

Boundaries—Yes, You Need Some

Not every fat person has boundary issues, but a whole lot of us do. We feel unworthy of love and protection in some fundamental ways. We compromise ourselves. We lack the confidence and self-esteem to stand up and say "go to hell" or even "no, you can't borrow five dollars."

How can you tell if you have boundary issues? Do you find yourself giving others your time, energy, or resources, and then resenting them? Do you feel over-extended or taken advantage of? Do you feel like you give more to other people than they give to you? Do you ever feel like you have to do things for the people in your life or they will abandon you? Do you ever find yourself doing things that you know are unsafe or reckless because someone wants you to?

If the answer to any of these is yes, then you're giving more of yourself than you really want to. It's time to turn that around.

I'm not going to try to teach a seminar on boundaries. I'm sure a quick search can yield many great resources that can help you develop healthy edges around yourself. If you suspect you have trouble with this, buy a book and start working through the exercises. In the meantime, the short form is: start practicing saying "no."

Here's a radical thought that spun my head around when I first heard it: "No" is a complete sentence. Seriously. Not only are you allowed to say it, but you don't have to explain why you said it. If someone is asking for your time, energy, or resources, it's up to you to decide whether to give them. If you choose not to, that's your choice, and you do not owe them an apology or your guilt.

You have to come first in your own life. Who else is going to put you first if you don't? If you keep working for others and not recharging yourself, do you think that might have a negative impact on you? It makes it harder to keep caring for others when you're an exhausted husk of a human being.

As you start learning to protect yourself, be aware that when you first start using a disused voice, it can come out all rusty and froggish. Over time we get better at it, more graceful, and the voice comes out naturally. It really helped me to understand that 1) I needed to keep practicing using my voice, and 2) if people reacted to it like it was too aggressive, it might have been. The words didn't always come out gracefully because it was so hard for me to force them out of my mouth.

If you find that you're upsetting those close to you with your new proactive stance about your availability, consider clueing them in. Tell them you're working on speaking up for yourself, and if it comes out badly you apologize, but you're not going to stop doing it. Then you can step back and let them work through their own crap about your changes. Other people's resistance to you changing is not a reason to stop changing. I mean, think about it—you're taking away their free ride. You're expecting the scales to balance in the relationship for a change. Of course they're going to be a bit grumpy about it.

Stand your ground, be as gentle as you can in your new firmness, and learn to defend yourself. You deserve it.

Choosing When to Come Out as a Former Fatty

It's hard to know when to tell people I used to weigh a hundred pounds more than I do now. When I was in the process of losing the weight, everyone I knew was having to deal with a different Freya. I was often unrecognizable to people I'd known for years. So many of my conversations began with a discussion of my weight or the change in my appearance. All of my interactions with people felt a bit like I was being seen through layers of gauze—Skinny Freya laid on top of Fat Freya, and the person I was talking to being a bit off-balance as a result.

When Skinny Freya got to make a new friend who had no idea Fat Freya had ever lived, it was like a breath of fresh air. I found it incredibly peaceful to have a new friend who related to me just as I was now, not this confusing amalgamation of past and present.

Then there's boys. Do I really want to tell a new man I'm dating that I used to be huge? Wouldn't that perhaps make him run for the hills, before that fat chick trapped inside me ate her way back out?

Deciding when to come out as a former fat person is a tough call. We want to be seen as who we are by those we're close to. We want them to know the real us, and the fat to thin adventure is part of who we are. But that period before they know can feel like a safe honeymoon away from reality, one I was sometimes reluctant to let go of.

One guideline is to ask yourself, "Are we at the intimacy point where they could be legitimately mad that I didn't share this important thing about myself?" or in other words, "Am I starting to feel like I'm hiding something by not sharing?" If the answer is no, then you can tell if you want to, not if you don't. If the answer is yes, it's probably best to bite the bullet and get the disclosure over with as casually as possible. You don't have to get out photos or anything.

How hard do you want to make it for people to find out you used to be fat without you telling them? Do you untag all the fat pictures on Facebook? Do you erase that person like she never lived? Do you get a new driver's license photo and try not lying about your weight on it for the first time ever?

These are all really personal questions. The answer will depend on how private you are, how much it helps you to have others know about your journey, and your approach to intimacy and relationships. Sometimes it will come down to your mood. I've had a great time telling total strangers, like the girl helping me at Nordstrom, about my losses, when I wasn't sharing with someone I was dating. I've never regretted telling someone, but I have enjoyed the quiet oases of privacy when they occurred.

It hurt me, a lot, to put up the start-to-finish photo gallery on Facebook. I had been one of the untaggers. I had a photo album up on a weight loss site, but that was just for people in the same boat I was. Making that gallery publically available as part of book promotion provoked a medley of emotions: humiliation, relief, anxiety, and pride.

Once it was done, I got used to it. Hopefully you'll be able to find a good balance in your own journey, between protecting your privacy and your right to remake yourself, and your need to connect to others in a transparent way.

Sex

I approve of sex. Quite a lot, actually. But before I talk about the general awesomeness of sex, I'd like to just make a couple cautionary notes.

If it's been a while since you were sexually active, please remember to be gentle with yourself. Using one's fat to insulate one's self from relationships is a protective mechanism. When you remove the fat, you're like a turtle without its shell for a while. If you need to take things really slow, do so. If you need to go on a couple dates, freak out, and then not date for a month while you think things over, do that. Remember that you're the only one who can safeguard your delicate exposed skin.

Also, if it's been a while since you were dating new partners, you'll need to get brushed up on the latest safer sex protocols. Find out what the experts are recommending. Know how different things are transmitted and what your risk factors are. Get vaccinated for whatever you can. Remember that many fat people have deep-seated self-esteem issues. It is very easy to allow the desire for affection and attention to lead you away from what you need to do to keep yourself safe. No one's attention is worth unsafe sex. It's not really love if the price is putting your health at risk. If you're not sure about your motivations or practices, please find someone to talk to. Take good care of yourself, to make sure you are writing a happy ending to this story of your weight loss adventures.

Let's move onto the upside of sex, shall we? First off, it can help you maintain your weight loss. Scientists have figured out that sex and hunger are regulated by the same brain chemical. If you have regular sex and satisfy that appetite center it can help satisfy the desire for food as well. Let that be a lesson to you, kids: science says sex is good for you.

Getting thinner can have an amazing impact on one's sex life as well. Personally, I am more limber, energetic, enthusiastic, and feel more. I have a higher libido than I did when fat—I have more available energy and it's fun to burn some of it in bed. When I started having sex again after a long break, I called my body "my new sex toy." It felt dramatically different from the body I was used to having sex with. I kept finding myself thinking "let's see if I can do this!" And then I could.

I got a whole new kind of orgasm. There's less belly in the way or something, and some sexual positions result in fireworks that never could before. Keep an open mind. Play around. Get on top and pretend your boobs and belly skin aren't bouncing.

You might be surprised by how amazing things can get.

XII. REENTRY AND MAINTAINING FOR LIFE

Never trade what you want most for what you want at the moment.

When to Stop

At some point during my weight loss journey, I had a blinding flash of inspiration: just because I got up to 235 doesn't mean I have to settle for 150. What if I could actually lose all the weight I wanted to, and get to a weight that feels right for me? My commitment and my food plan gave me that control, and I went down to 135 before I called "goal."

How do you decide where goal is? It's a surprisingly hard thing to figure out.

Several factors weigh in on the "keep losing" side:

- It's addictive watching the numbers on the scale go down every week. We get giddily hooked on being able to post a loss on our tickers online and tell our friends we're now down 75 pounds, etc. The idea of having the scale show the same number week after week, or even fluctuate *up* a couple pounds, is nowhere near as attractive.
- We might have an idea in our minds that we want to be a size four before we stop.
- We might be chasing the weight we were in high school, when we got married, or some other significant benchmark.
- We might want to lose to a little below where we want to end up, so we have a buffer for maintaining.
- It's incredibly important to achieve the number we set as "goal" months before, so we know we've accomplished what we set out to do. Stopping three pounds short of goal because we're exhausted and frustrated will be selling ourselves short in the long run. We need to hang in there until we can yell our success to the rooftops.
- We are terrified to lose the structure of the diet we've been on and experience the endless ocean of food choices represented by maintenance.

Several factors weigh in on the "call it goal" side:

- It turns out we like our body with a little bit of curviness to it, and want to remain a little soft around the edges.
- Our body resists the number we dream of, telling us that it won't be able to maintain that number realistically and healthily. It's better to stop at a number that actually works for our body, metabolism, and lifestyle, so we can remain there without having to live on celery sticks.
- We've achieved a healthy BMI.
- While it's tempting to stay with the addictive pleasure of a decreasing weight, we recognize that we're already healthy and should enjoy that.
- We choose not to believe our "fat goggles" which tell us we're still gigantic, and instead believe the number on the scale and the feedback of others that we're at a good weight.
- We set our "goal" number months before, and now that we're lower we find it's not where we actually want to be. We feel good, our body feels good, and we adjust the goal number to something that matches our experience of our body now.
- We have a lot of loose skin cluttering up our ability to tell what's really going on. We decide to stay at goal for a year or two, allowing our skin to catch up and shrink down. Then, if we still want to take off five or ten more pounds, we can do it later.

How do we choose? There are certainly a lot of competing ideas above. One way to decide is based on BMI. While BMI is a rather blunt instrument (one size fits all never actually does), if you set your goal so you're just inside healthy (no longer overweight), you're probably not underweight no matter what your bone structure.

Another way is to check in with your doctor. Your doctor will hopefully have a good mix of information about you, based on your weight, blood pressure, overall physique, cholesterol levels, age, etc. They can work with you to select a goal weight that's a good mix of low enough to be healthy and high enough to maintain.

Friends and family can be a good source of information, but only if they actually have a healthy relationship with food and their weight, and aren't jealous of you. When I looked around at my social world I realized I didn't actually know these people. Almost everyone I knew was either overweight or underweight, or had an eating disorder, refused to eat green vegetables, only ate once a day, or had some other overt food weirdness that ruled them out as having a healthy vantage point. I believe that people with a healthy relationship with food and weight exist, but I don't have them in my close circle of friends. If you're lucky enough to have some around you, ask them what they think of your current weight and planned goal. They'll have good input.

Don't be afraid to adjust your goal as you get closer to it, especially if it's been many years since you've been that weight. You might decide to raise or lower the number once you see how it wears on your body now. Even this can be challenging, as I like my naked body better with a little more fat rounding out the curves and loose skin, but I like myself better smaller in clothes. This also changes over time as I add muscle and my skin shrinks. Seeing how it wears on my body now still gives me conflicting input.

Whatever you do, don't quit before success. Make sure you know you've done what you set out to do before you stop. Give yourself a gigantic win to sustain you through maintenance. It helps a lot to know that you did it.

You did it.

Have a Plan

You're going to need a food plan. We settled the question earlier about whether you have issues with food. If you gained weight because your doc put you on a medication or you have a health condition and for no other reason, then your doc has given you a food plan to take the weight back off and you're not reading this book. If you were fat for any other reason, you have issues with food.

Having issues with food means that you don't get to go back to "eating normally" now that you're at goal. First off, go to Red Robin or Outback and see what our culture thinks eating "normally" looks like. It's pretty disgusting. Huge portions of fried, sauce-drenched, carb-laden food, with a giant slab of sugar to finish it off. You are not going back to that kind of normal now, because that will mean being fat again. Quickly.

Nor are you going back to some kind of normal that involves eating whatever you want. You cannot trust yourself. You are *not to be trusted*. Trusting your food impulses makes you fat. Period.

Does this mean you can't listen to your body at all? Yes and no. Your body will still be a worthless liar on many, many occasions. Other times it will be giving you genuinely useful feedback that you need more fuel for your current exertion levels. How can you tell the difference? If you've spent the day on the sofa and it says you need cheesecake or Doritos, it's a worthless liar. If you've spent the day splitting firewood and it says it would really, really like some plain grilled chicken breast, maybe it's short on fuel and you should give it some.

However, no matter how good you get at sorting out the liar from the good information, listening to your body should still comprise only about 3% of your food decisions. The rest need to come from a solid, reliable food plan.

Yes, you must have a food plan. Without one, the world of choices will swamp you. You will regain the weight you lost, and probably add some more. To provide a little mathematical proof for this: if you eat a hundred calories a day more than you burn, you will gain fifty pounds in five years. As a dieter, I'm pretty confident you know exactly how teensy a hundred calories is. One cup of vanilla ice cream is 300. A small McDonald's fries is 230. Two double-stuffed Oreos are 140. One piece of garlic bread is 170. One cup of white rice is 205. Three ounces of rib eye are 174. A typical protein bar has about 210. One medium apple is 95.

You get my point, right? One tiny snack here or there, one extra piece of bread, one more serving of dinner or scoop of ice cream, and you're heading right back to fatness. Do this on a daily basis and it's inevitable.

So let's don't do this on a daily basis. Instead, you need to figure out how many calories you burn and what intake level lets you maintain your weight. The basic concept is simple. When calories in = calories burned, you maintain. If your weight goes up, you drop your calories. Logging everything you eat is essential as you figure this out.

The nuances are anything but simple. There is no magic food plan that is going to work for everyone. Some people like more meat protein, or are vegan. Some handle dairy well, others find that cheese sticks to their hips like glue no matter what they do. Some thin people regularly snack on fruit and yogurt, while others find that the sugar in fruit makes it hard to stay on an even keel with their blood sugar. Some people can manage small portions of grains, while others find they trigger a feeding frenzy.

With all this to figure out, where do you start? Start with the guidance from the diet you've been on. Hopefully it's a doctor-recommended and well-conceived plan, and provides a gradual transition and long-term maintenance plan. Give that a shot. Log your food and weight. Notice what happens. If you go up, cut portion sizes, carbs, or calories. If you keep losing, increase portion sizes, carbs, or calories.

Remember that a pound of fat represents 3500 calories. So if you ate one Oreo yesterday and today you're up two pounds, those things are not causally related. You did not eat 7000 extra calories yesterday. You need to step back a bit and look at whole weeks, or even a few weeks, to know what's really happening. If you're eating 100 extra calories a day it takes a whole month for that to show up as a pound on the scale. But if you're eating 500 too many each day, you'll have that pound in just a week.

The basic idea with a transition plan should be to gradually reintroduce some foods that have been off your list, and gradually increase the calories you're taking in. Keep the focus on gradual. *Gradual.* Seriously. Add one new food at a time, and stick with it as your only new food for a few days. See what happens to your energy levels, mood, allergy reactions, and most importantly, your cravings for other foods. If it works well for you, you can keep it and incorporate it into your food plan. If it sends you into any kind of a tailspin, eliminate it from consideration for at least a few months, if not forever.

One of the things that was hardest for me to figure out was that I needed a particular ratio of protein and carbs in any meal, in order to not get all wonky. I mean, if I'm having carbs, I need a certain ratio of protein to balance it out. I can eat all the protein I want and my body never gets tired of it, but carbs are problematic. I could eat an energy bar with 14 grams of carbs and close to no protein and get all spun out, or a bar with 24 grams of carbs and 14 grams of protein and be totally fine. It took a lot of trial and error to realize that it wasn't grain that was the problem, it was the grain to meat ratio. You will have your own quirks. This involves a lot of science.

Things will change over time, as your body adjusts to its new way of eating. At first, any carbs at all were very challenging for me. Later, I could eat carbs as long as there was two to three times as much protein in the meal. After that, I got to where it could be 24/14 and I was fine. That took several months of maintenance, though.

What does a good food plan look like? Healthy eating, sustainable habits for your lifestyle, and a small amount of flexibility for adapting to changing circumstances.

Healthy eating: for most people, this means small meals throughout the day. Shopping the perimeter is important, so you're eating fresh whole foods. A solid base of protein and vegetables, with some grains, dairy, and fruit. It's going to involve portion control to keep calories within bounds. It will likely involve cooking most of your food, as getting low-fat healthy options in restaurants or frozen is challenging and expensive. If you don't know what healthy eating looks like, consult with a nutritionist or do some reading. Buy the South Beach cookbooks. Eat scary vegetables like kale and parsnips. Learn to cook fresh food with olive oil. Push yourself to broaden your horizons and take in the best nutrition you can.

Sustainable habits: your plan needs to work with your lifestyle. If you travel half your life for work, your food plan will look very different from that of someone who works from home. If your job and commute keeps you away from your house for fourteen hours a day, it will look different from the plan of someone who is only gone for nine and can cook a fresh dinner every night and have the leftovers for lunch the next day.

You have to work around housemates who eat your food, scheduling conflicts, refrigeration options, food breaks at work (clean rooms present quite the challenge for people trying to eat many small meals!), budget, etc. Being realistic about available time, energy, and funds is critical. However, no matter what your constraints, you *will* be able to devise a food plan that lets you maintain your weight.

Flexibility: your plan needs to have a little room for flexibility, but not too much. Some people will want to leave room in their calorie budget for the occasional piece of cheesecake. Others will know that any sugar will send them into a lengthy binge and their food plan will never allow it.

Note that "flexible" doesn't mean "this food is free because I have to live a little sometimes." You know that thing that you hear thin people say sometimes? "I had a small salad for lunch so I could save room for dinner out" or "I'll be paying all week for this dessert." It sounds like a foreign language to me, but what they mean is simple. They take in a certain number of calories on a daily/weekly basis to maintain their weight. If they go over it for a special indulgence they make up for it by restricting their calories elsewhere. Build in the flexibility you can handle, but make sure to compensate for it elsewhere.

I'm six months into maintenance and still figuring out what my food plan looks like. I've got the basic structure hammered out. It works well for me to eat about six times a day. My current lifestyle allows me to spend an afternoon cooking a couple times a week, prepping a bunch of food. My meals are pretty much all the same: 225-250 calories of lean protein and vegetables, with perhaps some yogurt, cheese, or a tiny amount of grain. I supplement with protein bars when I want a carb hit. I do not have a tight grasp on how much I can indulge when at a party or restaurant, and that's what I blame for having put a few pounds back on. I'm continuing to work with my plan, because flexibility is still troublesome for me.

Sorting out your plan is going to be incredibly difficult. This is where most dieters fail. They get to goal and relax all self-control. They figure they've done it, now is the easy part.

That thinking will put you in an early grave. Maintenance is the hard part. Losing the weight was easy by comparison. However, you lost the weight, so you know you're a freakin' rock star already. You can absolutely do this.

Commit to yourself. Commit to your health. Experiment, collect data, notice your reactions to foods, learn about nutrition and your body.

Write down your plan and follow it. Weigh every week. If your weight stays within your maintenance range (I set a five-pound range as my window), keep following it. If your weight goes above or below your range, tweak it.

You can do this. It may be the hardest thing you've ever done, but you can do it. Your goal jeans are worth it. Stand on the steps of

Tara and scream to the heavens, "I will never wear elastic waist bands again!"

Then go log your food and stick to your plan.

Avoid Triggers—Slow Testing

As I mentioned above, slow scientific study is essential for transitioning off your strict weight-loss diet into a lifetime food plan. You need to introduce one new thing at a time. This allows you to identify your triggers—foods that induce cravings or bingeing.

Some triggers are straightforward things. Roasted salted nuts are a trigger for me. They make me want to eat vast quantities of roasted salted nuts. Give me a container of the Kirkland fancy nut mix from Costco with the macadamias in it, and I'll keep filling my bowl until the container's gone or out of my house. It's the classic "one is too many and a thousand isn't enough" addiction response. Guess what I do with roasted salted nuts? Avoid them.

Some triggers are odd, sideways things. For me, fruit makes me want to eat other carbs. It doesn't send me into a fruit binge. Instead, strawberries in a fruit smoothie can make me desperately crave white rice and Fritos for the rest of the day. Oddly enough, the straight up sugar in a protein bar doesn't give me any trouble, but I think that's because it's paired with enough protein to ground out my reaction to it.

People can be triggered by sugar in general, or just pound cake. They can be triggered by fried food in general, or just mozzarella sticks.

You may be very surprised by what your triggers are. I found that bacon didn't trigger me in the slightest. I could eat two pieces and leave the rest of the platter alone on the buffet. It's not that I don't love bacon, I do. For the entire nine-year period I was vegetarian, when asked what my favorite foods were I would reply "bacon and avocados." So I was sure it would be an issue for my self-control. Nope.

These surprises are why we do slow scientific study when reintroducing foods. Eat a new food, then monitor your reaction for the rest of the day. Cravings? A rash, headache, or stuffy nose? Fatigue? Overeating? These are all bad signs. Since you've introduced only one food, you know what food to attribute them to.

If you had a mild reaction, you might wait a couple days and then try that food again, just to be sure. You could try it at a different time of day, or in combination with other foods. If it's a strong reaction, you probably want to dust off the debris from the binge and put that food in the "no thank you" category for a lengthy or permanent time-out.

If you seem okay after the first time of trying it, try it again for the next few days. Keep monitoring your reactions. All green lights? Then it's approved to be part of your maintenance food plan.

Now you can try adding one more food.

This process is very like allergy testing with an elimination diet. You've been on an elimination diet, removing all the foods that cause you to gain weight. Since your system's all cleared out, take advantage of this opportunity to really see how you react to things. It might be a bit of a pain to separate your testing of wheat, marinara sauce, cheese, and pepperoni into separate days. But if you just eat a piece of pizza instead and find it messes you up, you haven't learned all that much. You learned not to eat pizza, sure. But what if it's the cheese and not the rest of it that's the problem? If you'd tested cheese alone, you'd know you can eat pizza without cheese instead. Or what if it's the wheat? You might find that pizza made on a spelt crust is no trouble for you.

Bear in mind that your reactions may change over time. The Medifast diet was so low carb that I was especially hair-trigger in my reactions to all carbs when first transitioning off it. That has settled down a lot six months later. Doesn't mean I don't keep an eye on them, but they're not as firmly in the "trigger" category as they were at first.

One new food at a time. *Science!*

Log Your Food and Tweak Your Plan

In maintenance, the learning never ends. You will change over time. Your body will change over time. Your lifestyle and circumstances will change. You may exercise more or less, or just differently.

All these things can cause you to gain or lose weight. You have set a maintenance window, and you weigh at least once a month (or get into your goal jeans), so you know when you're off track.

Once you know you're off track, you tweak your plan. If you've been logging your food all along, you can quickly assess the situation with all the information you need. You can look at total calories, carbs, and fat. You can check out the carb to protein ratio, or the percentage of calories from fat. If you haven't been logging your food, start immediately. Every bite gets entered and counted. Once you have the information you need, you might spot the problem in just a couple days.

Then tweak your plan. This will be an ongoing process, perhaps a lifetime one. We keep learning. We get cocky, thinking "sure, I can handle a little fried food," and then discover we're getting fatter by the week. Or we change, and discover that we can handle a little fried food on occasion. It's an utterly personal process.

Keep exploring your feelings about and reactions to foods. Keep investigating the emotions or situations that make you overeat or want to overeat. Perhaps your food plan involves "avoid bars" because of the temptation towards beer and bar food, or "avoid movie theaters" because you can't handle the smell of popcorn.

Remember that your food plan is a living, breathing thing. Let it keep evolving as you do.

When You're Up, You Work

Unless you've suddenly become a totally new person through losing some weight, your weight will go up. It will slowly creep up, a half-pound every couple weeks. It will jump up after a little carb breakdown at Olive Garden. It will come like a thief in the night, and before you know it, you'll be making excuses for the number on the scale and pretending you're just not "in the mood" for jeans today.

It will happen.

When it does, you work.

It's hard work, and there are lots of possible ways to go about it. You'll need to experiment to find out what strategy is going to work for you for course-correction. But all roads to maintaining your weight begin with:

Step 1: Reality. Fighting the denial is half the battle. Here are some of my favorite ways to try to duck the reality of the scale:

- I've been exercising—I'm just retaining water.
- I'm pre-menstrual—I'm just retaining water.
- I'm menstrual—I'm just retaining water.
- I ate too many carbs recently—I'm just retaining water.
- I'm constipated—I'm just retaining... you get the idea.
- I didn't get enough sleep. If I slept longer, I'd be down another couple pounds by the time I woke up.
- It's all the extra muscle I've been building with all that exercise.
- It's just a natural fluctuation; it'll go back down again.
- It's just a pound or two.
- I'll deal with it tomorrow (or after the weekend, after that event with the buffet...).
- Maybe my body isn't meant to maintain so low. I look good curvy.
- My man still thinks I'm sexy, what do I care if I'm up a couple pounds?

I've had each and every one of these thoughts in the last week alone. It's kind of impressive how many different ways my brain can attack this one problem: an indisputable number on the scale. And yet, I dispute it!

The first step on the road to maintaining your weight loss is admitting the truth. You have to weigh every week. And then you have to actually admit the truth of the number on the scale. Admit reality into your mind, so you can take action.

Step 2: Information. You need to know what the problem really is. Have you been logging your food? Great! Now you can assess the track record of what you've been eating. Too many carbs? Too much fat? Too many snacks? Too much eating out? Too little exercise? Giving in to a trigger food? Drinking too much alcohol? Not enough vegetables?

You're a smart person. You knew enough about nutrition to lose the weight in the first place. You know the basic equation that when calories in > calories out, you gain weight. It's not rocket science. You are fully capable of identifying the problem with a little careful examination.

If you haven't been logging your food, start. You might be shocked to see how those little nibbles here and there add up. You might identify something you've been eating that just isn't worth the carb hit you're taking for it. Logging your food is essential.

You might also consider one of those exercise tracker armband thingies, that records your heartbeat and calories burned throughout the day. Most people vastly over-estimate the number of calories they burn through exercise. After exercise, they say "I just burned 1,000 calories so now I can eat 800 more and still lose weight." But what if you actually only burned 500 and you're eating 600 a day more than you burn overall? Still gaining weight, even after visiting the gym.

What if you're not sure where the problem is? Ask someone else. Share with them what you've been eating in a typical day, and what your exercise plan looks like. Ask them for their insights. And then don't get angry at them—remember, you asked.

Information is your ally. Collect all you can.

Step 3: Make a plan. What are you going to do to turn things around? What are you willing to give up? What are you unwilling to give up that you have to give up anyway? You could:

- Go back on your old diet, the one you used to lose all the weight
- Go back to a modified version of your old diet, some intermediate stage of the transition plan
- Adjust your current food plan to reduce calories or carbs
- Cut out beer and desserts
- Cut out carbs
- Eliminate snacks
- Only eat every 3 hours no matter what
- Eat every 3 hours no matter what
- Exercise 5 days a week
- Stop bingeing
- Stop eating for emotional reasons: boredom, anxiety, grief, anger, loneliness
- Avoid restaurants and frozen food, cooking your own meals instead
- Weigh and measure everything you eat

-Only you can know where you are off track. You've identified the problem, now choose a solution. Make a plan. Write it down.

Step 4: Commit. Right now, today, get back on track. You don't have tomorrow, you only have today. Tomorrow doesn't exist anywhere. Tomorrow is what let us all get so damn fat in the first place. Tomorrow is the word that lets people get so fat they can't walk and their ass grows into the fabric of their sofas— "I'm too tired to get up today, but tomorrow I'll start exercising and eating less fried chicken." No, you won't.

Do it now. Commit to your plan. You are worth it. You are worth changing your life forever. You are better than your habits and your past. You can choose to change, and you can succeed at becoming a different person.

Now. Today. Commit.

Step 5: Work. Yeah, it sucks. Yes, you'd rather lie in bed and eat bonbons. So would we all. That doesn't matter, though. Because little jeans and being picked up when your man hugs you and the joy of moving around in a fun little body is worth some work.

It's worth it.

Now do it.

Try to Relax

Now the hardest part of all, trying to relax. For my final message to you, I would like to assure you that you are not going to wake up the morning after eating one tater tot and weigh a hundred pounds more.

Not even if you ate two tater tots.

We have so much fear of ending up fat again. We were miserable there. We didn't know just how miserable until we lost the weight and remembered what it was like to live fully. Now we know just how much we have to lose.

Fat doesn't come back overnight. When we regain the weight we've lost, we do it slowly. It actually takes a fair amount of hard work. We have to overeat consistently, and we have to maintain our denial. If you keep crushing your denial like a bug, by getting on the scale and checking your goal jeans for muffin top, you're not going to put on fifty pounds without noticing.

You will notice. It will start slow, with a couple pounds here or there. You have the tools and the commitment to stop it at that point.

You can relax a little bit. Want to try a bite of someone's crème brûlée? Okay. As long as sugar isn't a general trigger for you, the world will not end. Want to have a beer? Fine, go right ahead. Log it, adjust your food plan for the rest of the day or week to accommodate it, and enjoy it.

Gained a couple pounds? No need to panic. Just do what you need to do to take it back off.

Yes, it feels like there is a fat person squished inside your skinny skin, bursting at the seams, just waiting for one potato chip to open the zipper and let her pop back out. This is not actually true. One moment of inattention, one slip in your vigilance, does not result in instant obesity.

Thinking it does is part of that all-or-nothing thinking that gets us into trouble anyway. One potato chip is not an excuse to eat the whole bowl and then head to the minimart for more. Have a chip. Enjoy it. Let it be okay to eat the one and stop.

Wake up the next morning and discover you're still slim and lovely. Take a deep breath. Open your arms to the wide adventure of your life. It's waiting for you.

What are you going to do now?

KEEP IN TOUCH!

Thank you for reading Suddenly Skinny! To stay in touch, please visit facebook.com/SuddenlySkinny, Twitter @SuddenlySkinny, or SuddenlySkinny.blogspot.com.